Dedicated to all the sufferers of any mental health issue and their loved ones, and to those working tirelessly across all spectrums around the world to bring a better understanding and awareness of mental health issues through research, support and treatment.

By openly talking about mental health, we can pull the trigger on mental illness.

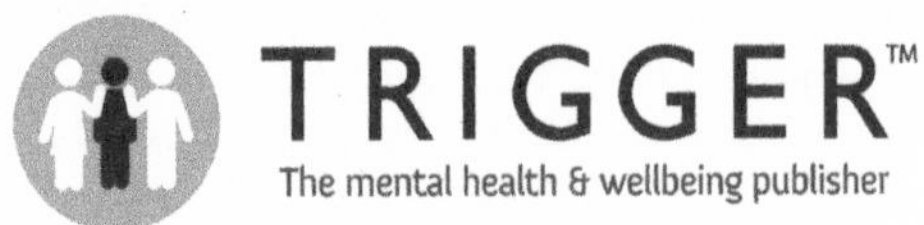

www.triggerpublishing.com

Thank you for purchasing this book.
You are making an incredible difference.

Proceeds from all Trigger books go directly to The Shaw Mind Foundation, a global charity that focuses entirely on mental health. To find out more about The Shaw Mind Foundation, visit **www.shawmindfoundation.org**

MISSION STATEMENT

Our goal is to make help and support available for every single person in society, from all walks of life. We will never stop offering hope. These are our promises.

Trigger and The Shaw Mind Foundation

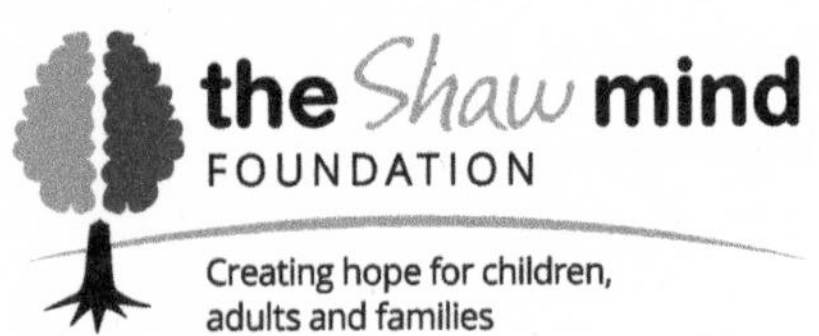

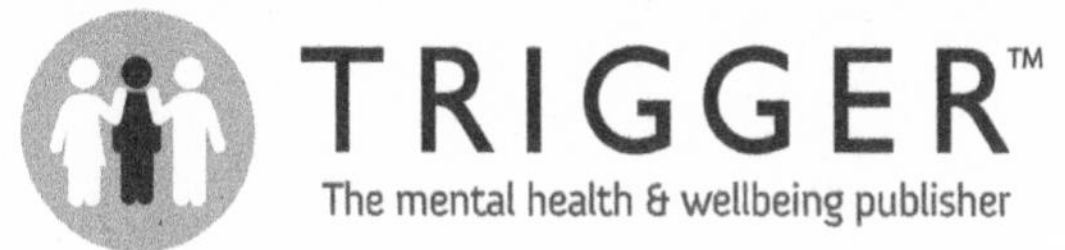

www.triggerpublishing.com

Postpartum Depression & Anxiety

The Definitive **Survival and Recovery Approach**

By Sonya Watson & Kathryn Whitehead

Trigger Press is proud to introduce this unique and inspiring self-help book. Written by a woman who has suffered from severe postpartum depression and a leading clinical psychologist, it provides simple yet highly effective self-help methods to help you overcome postpartum depression and anxiety.

THE AUTHORS

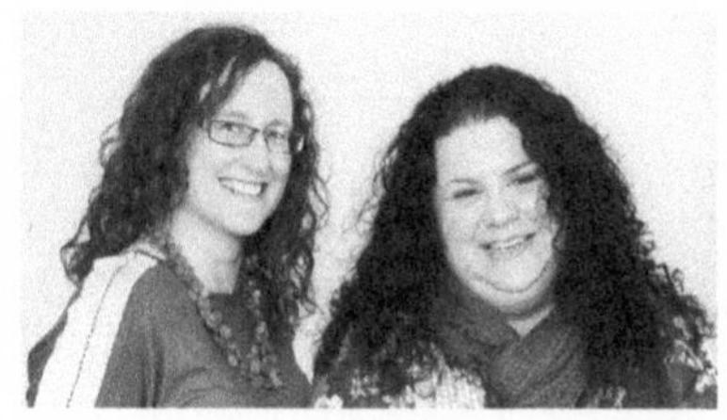

Sonya Watson is a mum of two and the Coordinator / Facilitator for PND Canterbury. After suffering with and recovering from postpartum depression, Sonya now uses her personal journey to inspire, educate and support others in the Canterbury region.

Kathryn Whitehead (MA (dist), PGDipClinPsych, MNZCCP) MNZCCP is a Clinical Psychologist who has worked for ten years at the South Island Regional Mothers and Babies Inpatient Service in Christchurch, New Zealand. Specialising in Acceptance and Commitment Therapy alongside attachment theory and intervention, Kathryn cares about helping clients, infants and their families build strong, connected and compassionate lives and relationships.

First published in Great Britain 2018 by Trigger Press

Trigger Press is a trading style of Shaw Callaghan Ltd & Shaw Callaghan 23 USA, INC.

The Foundation Centre
Navigation House, 48 Millgate, Newark
Nottinghamshire NG24 4TS UK

www.triggerpublishing.com

British Library Cataloguing in Publication Data

A CIP catalogue record for this book is available upon request from the British Library

ISBN: 978-1-78956-040-4

This book is also available in the following Audio and e-Book formats:

MOBI: 978-1-78956-043-5
EPUB: 978-1-78956-038-1

Cover design More Visual Ltd

Typeset by Fusion Graphic Design Ltd

Project Management by Out of House Publishing

Printed and bound in Great Britain by Clays Ltd, Elcograf S.p.A.

Paper from responsible sources

CONTENTS

Introduction 1

PART I SONYA'S STORY

Chapter 1: Who Knew It Would Be So Hard to Get Pregnant? 6
Chapter 2: Getting Caught up in Fear 11
Chapter 3: 'The Stress Was Awful ... But I Still Didn't Want to Ask for Help' 17
Chapter 4: The Biggest Baby in Wairau 23
Chapter 5: 'I Looked at My Baby, and I Felt Nothing' 27
Chapter 6: The World's Worst Mum 36
Chapter 7: Pretending Everything Was OK 43
Chapter 8: The Hurricane Was Building 48
Chapter 9: 'Postnatal Depression, Here's a Website Go Look at It' 52
Chapter 10: 'They Told Me My Little Boy Was Going to Die' 57
Chapter 11: Letting Go of the Mask 68
Chapter 12: Devon's Story 73
Chapter 13: The Healing Road 82
Chapter 14: You Are Not Alone 89

PART II Pullingthe**trigger**™

Section 1: Balancing the Impossible 93
Section 2: Before You Start ... Stop! 96
Section 3: Where Does It Hurt? 104
Section 4: What Is This About? Some Information about Perinatal Mental Health 115
Section 5: Finding a Direction to Go 126
Section 6: Making Space: Willingness and Acceptance 135
Section 7: Becoming Aware 142
Section 8: Becoming a Soup Mum and Making Space for Yourself with Your Thoughts 154
Section 9: The Even Bigger Picture: Finding a Space from Which to Act 170
Section 10: Making Your Move Again, and Again, and Again 181

Conclusion 205

Recommended Resources 211

WARNING: This book contains thoughts about the possibility of suicide.

A note on terms: In this book, we use the terms postnatal depression and postpartum depression interchangeably. In the US, the term postpartum depression is commonly used. But in telling her story, Sonya has talked about her postnatal depression – as is the norm in New Zealand.

We also refer to perinatal depression (or prepartum depression) referring to feelings of depression associated with pregnancy and childbirth. Antenatal depression refers to feelings of depression before childbirth occurs.

INTRODUCTION

WHO NEEDS A PERFECT MOTHER?

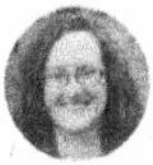

Kathryn: "Kids are like crack cocaine. When you're not with them, they're all you want. When you've got them, they're never enough!" These are the words of my cousin, Dr Simon Adamson, whose wise words manage to capture some of the profound ambivalence of parenting.

As children, there are few things that we're so comprehensively misled about than parenting. And there are few things for which experience really is the only way of knowing what it's really like.

I used to say that babies don't come with an instruction manual. I was wrong. They do come with an instruction manual. The problem is that you've got to learn a whole new language in order to translate it: the language of cues.

Luckily you knew this language once in your life, and you'll know it again. It's just a matter of spending a lot of time getting to know your baby and figuring out their way of telling you things. You can read material online to give you an idea of what can help, but a lot of it is learning through trial and error. The only problem with learning this way is that you have to make mistakes. And often we're so invested in our babies that it's very difficult to allow ourselves to make mistakes.

It isn't a question of being perfect, but of being good enough. This idea comes from Donald Winnicott, a paediatrician, psychotherapist, and leading thinker in the attachment field. Winnicott talks about the importance of having a good enough mother. As theories about attachment relationships have developed, the process of "rupture and repair" (Siegel, 1999), has become a critical part of building secure attachments. It's a process where a parent does a less-than-perfect job which causes a rift in the relationship, but the child comes to learn that this can be repaired.

Let's pause for a moment and try a thought experiment:

Imagine a child with an absolutely perfect mother. Let's say this mother could meet the child's every need absolutely perfectly. Imagine the child never even needed to cry to show her something was wrong, she could just anticipate it.

Now fast forward a couple of years and imagine what that child would be like.

What would they be like at school? What would happen if that child had problems that their teachers and peers couldn't anticipate at all times? Would that child be very good at making friends?

What would that child be like as an adult if they expected every single person they met to know, without asking or doing any extra work, exactly what the child needed?

We've got a name for people like this – we call them narcissists.

Perfection is not an ideal developmental solution. A core part of our relationships is the process of rupture and repair. The parent gets it a bit wrong, the kid does their best, and then they come back together, sort it out, and reconnect. It's that kind of process that builds a strong and stable relationship.

What does this mean for you?

We're led to believe that working harder will always lead to more success. So, unsurprisingly, it's a great shock for many parents to discover that, no matter how hard they work, they can't control their babies. This is something that you have to prepare for as a new parent. And that's what this book is about.

Through Sonya's explanations and the information that I'll give you, you will learn to make space in your life for this new baby, and for all the opportunities and adventures that can come with the challenges they bring.

Don't blame your hormones!

One of the important things to learn about postnatal depression is that it's actually not caused by hormones. There's a myth out there that it's hormonal but actually the highest risk factor for getting postnatal depression is a lack of social support in close relationships.

If we look back in time and see how humanity has developed and how our brains have evolved over thousands of years, we can recognise that the context we have today is not ideal for having babies. Today, we are all siloed into similar-age cohorts. We go to primary school and we play with other kids in our year who are the same age as us. We go to high school and we only interact with children our own age. At university, you don't see so many older people, and you certainly don't have any contact with younger children.

It becomes quite hard for the old and the young to be together, and there are fewer opportunities for it. Children are also less likely to have siblings, which means the parents of the next generation have fewer opportunities to learn how to relate to young infants and babies. Parents and their own children are separated younger and younger which means that our exposure to the agony and the ecstasy of parenting has never been shorter.

This all shows that the environment that humanity evolved in – the one that supported us in becoming effective parents, able to nurture children who are ready to go out into the world with a sense of security – is different to the world we find ourselves in now. We probably evolved to live in a group of about thirty people with a real mix of young and old. We would have watched other people as they became parents, we would have held babies and discovered what they're all about, and we would have discovered that it takes inordinate amounts of patience!

If we look at traditional societies, the role of parenting is often done by the grandparents. The actual parents will pop in and out for breastfeeding and some of the care, but actually, as the youngest and fittest, they spend most of their time getting food for the tribe. This means the patience and wisdom of grandparents has played a really important role within human history in helping babies to develop optimally.

What does this mean for you?

If you're like most parents nowadays, you're probably sitting on your own reading this with your baby – who may be asleep (yeah, right!) – to find your social supports, you will probably have to go out of the home. Perhaps you will have moved to a bigger house recently to help you accommodate the new addition to the family. These things all make you more vulnerable.

So what does this mean for you and your journey – and what does it mean for your recovery? It means that getting a support circle is more important than ever before in your life. It gives you important opportunities to reconnect with people who have supported you, to maybe build bridges, and reconnect with your own parents if you can.

It also gives you a vulnerability. If your experience with your own parents has been less than ideal, it's going to be a challenge for you as you move into this new period of your life. You may start to see your own parents in quite a different light and recognise that most of the time, like all of us, they were just doing the best that they could. Even if sometimes that wasn't actually good enough.

So, welcome! I hope that this book gives you some helpful opportunities to embrace. I hope it will help you become the kind of parent you always wanted to be, the kind of parent you didn't even know existed!

PART I

SONYA'S STORY

CHAPTER 1

WHO KNEW IT COULD BE SO HARD TO GET PREGNANT?

Sonya: When I look back at my experience of postnatal depression, I realise I probably suffered from antenatal depression too. There were lots of red flags that, in retrospect, suggested I was already experiencing depression before Jack was born.

My journey really started in 2007, when I found out that me and my husband, Devon, were pregnant. We were in our early thirties and we'd been married for around a year and a half. Devon was in the Air Force at that stage and we lived on an air base in Woodbourne, Blenheim, New Zealand. It was quite a close-knit community and we enjoyed the lifestyle. We worked hard during the week and enjoyed socialising on Friday and Saturday nights (sometimes even Sunday nights too!). With its cafés and vineyards, Blenheim was a lovely place to live.

We knew we wanted a family and we'd been trying for what seemed like forever. (Who knew it could be so hard to get pregnant? Especially after all those warnings they give you in school!)

I remember going to see the doctor one day and I was feeling really sick but I couldn't quite work out why. After failing to get pregnant for so long it didn't even occur to me that it might have finally happened. But I did the test and it came back positive.

I remember feeling absolute joy that I was really going to have a baby. I had butterflies in my stomach. This is where my journey started ...

I knew Devon would be at home by the time I got back from my appointment – and so it seemed like the longest drive. I walked into our cute little cookie-cutter home in the married quarters, overlooking a vineyard, and I felt so nervous. I didn't even know why. This was what we'd been dreaming of and talking about for so long; we'd even talked about what we thought the baby would be like before we were even pregnant.

I walked through the house, still full of butterflies, looking for Dev. And there he was – ironing his blue uniform in the sunroom, the sunlight streaming through the large windows.

We fell into the normal sort of chat we had every day:

'How was your day?' he asked.

'It was good, thanks.'

We carried on like that for a little bit and then I said, 'I need to talk to you for a minute ...'

Dev had his back towards me as he was ironing. He turned around and walked up to me. 'What's up?' he asked.

I held up the pregnancy test and he started to cry. And then I started crying too. It was a magical moment, a realisation that this was where our family would begin.

Back then, we didn't really know anything. I suppose we were quite naïve in some ways. We hadn't thought about the issue of support at that stage. My parents and my sisters lived in Christchurch, roughly four hours south of Blenheim, and Devon's parents lived in a little farming town on the outskirts of the North Island called Pahiatua. To get to their place, we would have had to take a ninety-minute flight to Palmerston North, and then drive another half an hour to their place.

I knew that our air force family would be there for us and support us. But we were the first of our group of friends to go through this, so I found that quite hard. (As it was 2007, we weren't on Facebook and we definitely weren't using Snapchat back then.)

We hadn't thought about how bringing a baby into our perfect marriage and our perfect house would change things. You get used to seeing those glamorous magazines showing how amazing the whole experience is ... and how easy. But now I know how different the reality is.

When I look back, and when I talk about it now, I can see how badly the antenatal depression hit me. I just didn't realise it at the time. I'd never really experienced anxiety or depression in my childhood, except perhaps when my mum was diagnosed with cervical cancer in her early thirties. I was only ten or eleven at the time and I remember crying a lot in my bed at night. Her treatment took around a year, and we used to stay with our grandparents because we weren't allowed to go and visit her in the old Christchurch Women's Hospital. She was very, very sick.

One night, I hid behind the door and listened in on a conversation between Mum and Dad. I heard her say, 'I don't want to go through treatment. I just want to die.' I was horrified and devastated. This was my mum! I couldn't understand why she wanted to die but somehow I thought it was my fault. I don't know why I blamed myself – was it because me and my sisters had been naughty?

Perhaps I did experience some depression back then. I stayed off sick from school because I couldn't face it. There was a time when I had to go and stay at a friend's place and her mum drank a lot, so that was scary. But I didn't want to bother Mum and Dad because they were going through enough as it was. Dad was trying to work, and Mum was going through radiotherapy, so I found it really hard to talk about what I was going through.

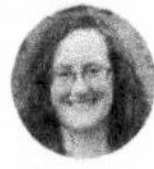

Kathryn: *Sonya's story shows how kids will usually attribute stressful situations to themselves, as they don't have the capacity to recognise that there are uncontrollable things that happen in life.*

But what did this mean for Sonya, as a mum-to-be?

Sonya's pregnancy would have had extra poignancy in the context of her awareness of her mother's mortality so early on. This would have played into her later fears of her baby dying and is just one factor that will have made her vulnerable.

Perhaps you have experienced trauma in your life too. Painful memories from childhood and relationships with our parents often resurface as we become parents ourselves. Sometimes we don't even realise these are memories; they may manifest as very strong emotions or a sense of déjà vu. Again, this can leave us vulnerable as we move into parenthood. Sometimes this can make us desperate to be nothing like our own parents, without having a sense of what we actually want to do differently. It might mean that we are flooded with fears and unresolved psychological issues that demand our attention when really, we'd prefer to be entirely focused on our baby.

Other times, having our own children can heal and integrate things in entirely unexpected ways. It's okay to tread carefully and be gentle to yourself as you embark on this journey, bringing with you all your history.

Our lives change in so many ways when we have children, and our relationships with our own parents often change too. Sometimes as we become parents ourselves, we discover that all those things that seemed so simple from a child's point of view are actually very challenging from the parent's perspective, and we begin to appreciate the challenges our parents faced. With this realisation comes gratitude.

Other times, parenthood can involve a painful discovery of what we might have missed as children. Perhaps the discovery of intense love and connection with a baby makes us realise that it was missing in our own childhood.

The attachment styles we develop as children, and our coping strategies for dealing with relationships, often persist into adulthood and other important relationships.

This can be a powerful dynamic. If we are aware of what's happening and can apply this understanding towards what matters to us in the long term, it gives us the opportunity to make change and choose how we want to parent our kids.

This shift in adult relationships, whether for the positive or negative, is another aspect of the profound change that occurs as we transition into parenthood.

Sonya: A lot of things happened the year my mum fell ill, and I just didn't know how to deal with them. I started my period, and though we'd talked about it in school a little bit, I felt lost because I didn't have Mum there to help me through it. I had to tell my friend's mum instead and it was awful because she could hardly afford sanitary pads. Life became a struggle, and I guess I really was experiencing little bouts of depression.

I didn't know a lot about depression. Mum and Dad never really spoke about it, and it wasn't spoken about at school. It wasn't discussed anywhere. I didn't learn about it until they briefly discussed it in one of my antenatal classes and even then, I didn't know enough until I started to struggle with my own postnatal depression.

CHAPTER 2

GETTING CAUGHT UP IN FEAR

Sonya: Mine was a classic pregnancy. I had morning sickness and cravings. It wasn't until we had a scan at twelve weeks that we met our midwife. I thought she was fantastic; she was really good and very understanding ... but I still felt like I couldn't ask her everything I wanted to ask. I had *a lot* of questions, but I didn't want to take up all her time. I didn't want to be a problem and I didn't want to sound like I didn't know what I was talking about. But of course I *didn't* know what I was talking about! How could I? I was a first-time mum.

I wish I had asked all those questions because I never found answers for them. Ten years down the line, as I was going over all of this again, I knew that I really needed those answers.

Baby looked fine in the twelve-week scan. He had feet, he had hands – although of course it was too early to know baby was a "he" back then. The nuchal fold at the back of his neck measured fine. (That meant the risk of Down Syndrome was low.) The brain was developing as it should be; everything was absolutely on track. As I continued through my pregnancy, all my blood tests came back fine, my urine samples came back fine, and my blood sugars were fine.

Devon and I had a good chat about it, and we decided that we wanted to find out the sex of the baby at our twenty-week scan. That was my controlling instinct kicking in – I like to be in control of my life – and we felt we needed to be organised for baby's arrival. We felt slightly anxious, even though it didn't really matter to us whether we were going to have a boy or a girl. I suppose I liked the idea of having a boy because I really wanted Devon to have a boy. I don't know why that was. Perhaps it was because I'd grown up without brothers and I liked the idea of our little boy taking on the family name.

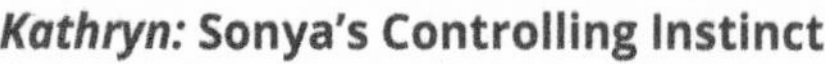

Kathryn: **Sonya's Controlling Instinct**

Control can work immensely well for us in our lives: it allows us to plan, organise, predict, and meet deadlines. Many highly competent and educated people are experts at control. Consider what society likes and how we praise children who have self-control. We can see how much our culture values organisation, efficiency, and competence.

By the time we become parents, we've often had a lifetime of learning that out in the real world, the more control we have, the better. The better our grades, the more we'll get paid, and the more other people will like us and tell us how great we are. We learn to pair safety and relaxation with this rule about "being in control". We lose touch with the fact that large amounts of our control are actually an illusion. If we were to recognise our daily vulnerability to accidents, the forces of fate, other people's cruelty, and how easily our life could be irrevocably changed in one instant, it would be utterly overwhelming.

It's psychologically helpful for us to feel in control. But becoming a parent is often a sure-fire way of opening ourselves up to the fact our control is not actually real. Our non-sleeping, colic-suffering, "What on earth is wrong with him / her" *baby gives us a very sudden immersion into the new reality. And we very quickly realise that our sense of control has been an illusion.*

Does this make us give up on our rules? No way! They're rules we've used for ages! And yet, they are also rules that can cause great suffering.

Is our capacity to feel relaxed and competent really dependant on being constantly in control? Is it possible that being in control could be part of the problem, rather than the solution?

Perhaps you could use this knowledge to help yourself let go a little and bring yourself back to what's actually happening in the moment you get this urge to assert control. You may find that information is available (which you are likely to have missed while you were so busy controlling) that can help you out.

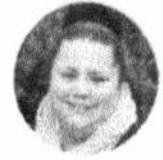

Sonya: We went for the scan at the hospital in Blenheim. With its tatty seats and décor, it looked a little bit old and tired. I told the receptionist who I was and why I was there and she just waved me over to the seats in a way that suggested she was a bit disinterested.

I'd had to drink lots and lots of water before the scan and my bladder felt as if it was bursting. By that stage, I was feeling a bit old and tired too! The pregnancy was just starting to feel more difficult. And when I look back, I can see that the twenty-week scan caused a lot of grief. But I went in, thinking everything would be fine ...

They were short-staffed that day so a first-year radiologist was on duty. And I didn't have any problem with that, in principle. Everything was going fine, he was scanning away, pointing out the hands and the feet. And then he said, 'Oh, we're having a boy!' That part was really exciting. We were thrilled!

And then he said, 'But ...'

As he said that, my heart started to race. I felt sick and I tried to work out what was happening. Had his little heart stopped? All sorts of questions flooded my mind.

But then the radiologist said, 'He's got cysts in his head. He's got cysts in his brain.'

I was devastated. Somehow, I held it in at first as the radiologist gave us more information. I held it in and held it in until I couldn't hold it in any longer. I cried as we walked out of the room.

When we got to the car, I rang Dad and said, 'It's a boy!' He was so excited for us, but I couldn't share the joy. I told him what we'd been told. He didn't panic, he just started looking it all up on the computer. He'd always been interested in the medical side of things. He should have become a doctor!

The radiologist had said they were choroid plexus cysts. And Google told us lots of different things that it could be and what it could look like. I later found out that lots of babies have these cysts in their brain, but you're just not told about them because they eventually disappear. But no one told us that at the time! And so our stress and the anxiety just ramped up. I thought our child was going to be born with brain development delays or grow up disabled. I was so worried, and a million questions went through my mind, all of them unanswered. Devon did a pretty good job of hiding it, but I knew he was just as worried as I was.

I didn't sleep a lot that night.

My midwife rang the next day to ask how I was doing. I told her I was fine, because that's what I do. That's how I react. That was the start of me putting the mask on and pretending everything was okay. She told me she'd just got the report from the radiologist and she congratulated me. But she didn't say anything else and I thought that was a bit strange.

So I said, 'What about these cysts?'

She said, 'How do you know about those?'

'The radiologist told us!'

The midwife sounded unimpressed. 'The midwife is supposed to know, and the doctors know, but they're not supposed to tell you because they do go away.'

I had to wait another eight weeks for another scan to see if they had started to disappear. The wait was excruciating. I tried not to think about it, but I couldn't stop worrying that I was going to have a miscarriage. That's when I really started to become quite anxious about the pregnancy. It got so bad that I would worry whenever I went to the toilet in case something happened. I'd never had a miscarriage before, but I was so scared about this little boy growing inside of me with cysts in his head.

I started to wonder how the doctors knew what sort of cysts they were. They must have seen them all the time, but I wanted to ask someone about it. Unfortunately, I didn't want to bother them. I knew I had to be brave and try to get on with things, but I felt sad. I kept asking myself why this was happening, not really believing that it was a fairly common occurrence. I didn't believe that there wouldn't be any consequences at the end of it. Babies are born and things are fine. If only the radiologist had explained it to me – if he'd told me what it was, and what the outcome would be – I would have been a lot happier.

Of course, when people would ask me how the pregnancy was going, I'd tell them it was all fantastic. Our families knew, but I didn't tell anyone else what had really been going on.

So we finally got to twenty-eight weeks for the scan and I was absolutely dreading it. Again, I had to drink litres and litres of water to inflate my bladder so they could see the baby better and then wait ... and wait ...

This time, the senior radiologist welcomed me in and told me to jump up on the bed. Straightaway, he said he needed to apologise. He told us he was really sorry for what had happened with the junior radiologist and said that he shouldn't have shared the information. He said the way he'd shared the information wasn't professional.

My midwife must have contacted him, so she'd done the best thing for me, but of course, I was still really pissed off. If I hadn't known about the cysts and we'd done another scan at twenty-eight or thirty weeks, I wouldn't have had the anxiety and the stress and the worry of what was happening. I wouldn't have panicked, wondering if our baby would be brain damaged ... or even if he'd be stillborn. I'd tried to push my fears away but wasn't able to.

The scan was clear. The cysts had gone.

The feeling of relief that washed over us both was absolutely massive, although I still couldn't quite let it go. I kept on saying, 'I hope you've got that right.' It took a while for it to really sink in, but when it did, I felt like I had a new lease of life.

Kathryn: Pregnancy Scans and Life in Your Hands

Conception and pregnancy are the first steps of a new, sudden responsibility for another being's life. What makes it all the more confusing is the fact that you don't know this baby yet. All you have is your dreams, fantasies, and worries about what might happen.

Part of becoming ready for parenthood is taking the time to get your head around the concept of this new-found responsibility before you actually hold the baby in your hands. (And if you're anything like me, you'll have a sudden and inexplicable fear you'll accidentally drop them!)

Factors such as significant health concerns for the baby in utero, severe morning sickness, maternal diabetes, and history of miscarriages can all leave you confronting the reality of life and death. Sometimes it means you have to come to terms with life and death earlier than other parents. The reality of not being in control hits hard, and often big fears emerge. This can make us vulnerable to anxiety and low mood.

It's really hard luck to miss out on getting used to the idea of a baby because you've had a complicated pregnancy or fertility history.

Giving yourself space to grieve for parts of the process that you missed out on is totally reasonable. You might need more opportunities to bond and connect with your baby because you didn't get the time to do it while you were pregnant. Be kind and patient with yourself as you do this. Recognising that you're getting caught up in fear about your pregnancy is the first step towards learning to live with it. That way you can work towards being the kind of parent you most want to be.

CHAPTER 3

'THE STRESS WAS AWFUL ... BUT I STILL DIDN'T WANT TO ASK FOR HELP'

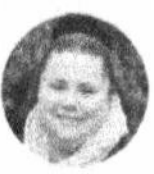

Sonya: Finally, the cysts had gone and I felt like I could start planning for our baby's arrival. I don't know anybody who buys a cot at six weeks, but I did! And from then on, I started buying nappies, wipes, powder and lavender bath soak. I just wanted to be organised. Soon our queen-size guest bed was absolutely covered with baby things.

It became a bit of an obsession. I was always buying baby things so that we wouldn't run out. I was like a hoarder of baby products – and my baby hadn't even been born yet! No one ever told me that you don't even use half of that stuff. But it didn't matter, because I was really excited.

A lot of red flags started popping up over the next couple of weeks, although I didn't recognise it at the time. It wasn't until I started to get really unwell that we realised that maybe something wasn't quite right.

Our world was rocked when Devon's best friend's wife, Shannon, passed away after battling multiple sclerosis. It was such a sad day. She had celebrated with us at our engagement party. We had shared some lovely times together, travelling to her home in Pahiatua. I always thought she was a cool person. She was kind and friendly and had a gorgeous family. It was heartbreaking watching her battle MS, and the hardest thing was knowing there was nothing we could do to fix it.

By the time she came to our wedding, she was in a wheelchair. A year or so later, she died. It really hurt to know she'd never get to meet our baby.

The due date was getting closer. Christmas was approaching, and our son was due at the start of January. It was hot in Blenheim, and I was getting pretty big! Walking was becoming harder and harder. But the whole family was coming for Christmas and I was very excited. We'd done the house up and we were all set.

But when I went out to meet Mum and Dad, I suddenly felt that something wasn't quite right.

I saw that Mum had been driving – and Mum never drove long distances. Dad got out of the car and just went straight into the house to sit down. That was really unlike him. Dad is always very busy and motivated. It was all a bit strange.

I followed him into the house. Everyone was very quiet. And then, as if to break the tension, Dad said, 'I need to tell you something ...'

Dad had had a stroke just a couple of days before coming to see us. Devon apparently already knew, but he'd kept it from me.

My world crashed. I felt sick and shaky. *My dad's not going to be around to see my baby!* I thought. It was really hard to take.

Dad had changed. He'd changed a lot. I had worked in palliative care and had seen stroke victims and seen cancer patients. I'd seen the aftereffects of big, life-altering illnesses. He didn't have a lot of feeling in his hands, he couldn't even switch the light on. He could still talk, but I could see he was exhausted all time. I'd never seen Dad so tired.

The worry set in straightaway. Now I know that anxiety was kicking in.

Over Christmas, I would lie in bed and my heart would start racing. I would over-think everything. I felt so nervous; what if he died in our house? What if he died on Christmas Day? What if, what if, what if ... I couldn't tell anyone about my worries. We didn't really speak about those kinds of things in our family. And I didn't want anyone else to worry.

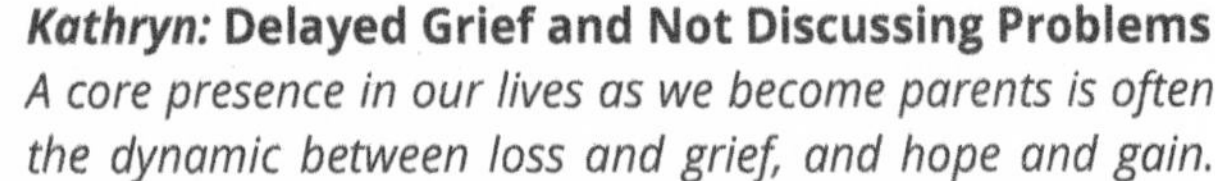

***Kathryn:* Delayed Grief and Not Discussing Problems**

A core presence in our lives as we become parents is often the dynamic between loss and grief, and hope and gain. You'll notice from Sonya's story that she experienced a lot of loss as she moved into motherhood. Because babies don't choose when they arrive and often neither do the parents, it's often the case that mothers can become depressed or highly anxious at times of great stress – and often when they have the fewest resources and the least capacity to cope. For example, people lose important members of their family while they're pregnant or when the baby is a newborn and they have no space to grieve.

You can see from Sonya's story that some of what she was struggling with was delayed grief: about her father's stroke, the loss of her good friend just before Jack's birth, and probably the loss of the fantasy pregnancy she'd had in her mind. There was no room for this grief in her life when it happened, and so she had to put it on hold. The difficulty with putting grieving on hold, whether you have a choice about it or not, is that it will come back to bite you. The grieving process has to happen in some way, somehow. And sometimes it will return even when we feel like your life doesn't have the space for it.

It's also possible that your grief at this time might not be about losing a particular person in your life. It might be more about losing a particular role or roles that you've played in life.

Becoming a mother can become all-consuming and thus we often lose track of the other parts of ourselves. Society and the people around us can lose track of them too and no longer see us as unique human beings, instead only seeing our roles as parents.

There can be other losses too: of our friends, social circles, sexual selves, or even the body we've always had. Bizarrely it can also seem to signal the loss of our childhood: children don't have children.

Sometimes there are subtler losses that can be just as challenging, particularly when we realise all of the things we've gained when we've had a new baby, a new life, a new role.

Be kind to yourself and take a moment here to notice what are the losses that you've experienced? What has it been like to lose these things?

Sonya: I was so worried about Dad. He seemed utterly beaten. And Mum was frustrated because he was sleeping so much, but I think it was because she was so stressed. I knew she had a history of anxiety and stress as well as bouts of depression (though I hadn't known what it was at the time), so it must have been really hard for her.

Everyone was really struggling, but none of us said, 'It's okay to have a cry,' or 'Let's talk about it.' We all just battled on in silence.

At least we were able to give Dad a great present: Devon and I had already decided we were going to call our little boy Jack Roger – Roger was my dad's name. He was over the moon when we told him.

We got through Christmas, despite my panicking that the stress would make the baby come early. But he didn't, and we just carried on waiting.

When Mum and Dad returned home, Dad had another stroke. I was so worried about him but I couldn't even travel down to see him. I wasn't able to fly or drive down to Christchurch, which is about three and a half hours away from where we lived.

I just tried to keep myself busy. I started doing endless cleaning and housework, emptying cupboards, and goodness knows what else – anything to keep myself busy. I didn't even think about what I was doing; I just started nesting. I wanted to make sure that everything was ready.

I really should have been resting though. Little did I know how much sleep I was going to miss out on over the next few months. But instead of taking the chance to sleep, I was labelling my herbs!

We decided to do a big "dump run" and clear all the clutter and Christmas wrapping out of the garage. So Devon loaded up the trailer, put a big blue tarpaulin over it, and tied it down with bungee cords. But as he was stretching, one of the cords snapped back right into his eye!

I heard this horrendous scream, but I thought it must have been the kids playing around. It was such a nice safe area, with lots of places for them to play, so I didn't think much of it. But then I saw him trying to crawl up the stone steps of the front porch. He could barely move. He was screaming in pain. I didn't think about calling an ambulance. I just knew I had to get him straight to hospital.

I'd never taken a trailer off a tow-bar in my life, but even at thirty-nine weeks pregnant, I learnt pretty quickly! I put a cold pack onto Devon's eye – I don't know why, but it seemed like the right thing to do. All the blood vessels in his eye had burst. There was blood all around his eye and all over his face.

At the hospital, they took us straight into a private room. They'd called the eye specialist who was out in Nelson, so they talked about flying Devon out there. But because I was due to have the baby any day, they brought the specialist to us instead.

No one could have prepared us for just how terrible it would be. The effects of the eye injury lasted for months and months – and Devon really suffered. He was so unwell that he couldn't dress himself or drive. He couldn't shower or go to the toilet without help. I had to help him get dressed, mow the lawn and do all those things he would normally have done. And of course it wouldn't normally be a problem, except for the fact that I was so heavily pregnant and I was tired.

The stress was awful, and I wasn't sleeping very well. I was getting more and more anxious about how the birth was going to go. What was I going to do? How was I going to cope when Devon was so ill? I couldn't even drive to the supermarket, I was that sore.

I sat down with Devon and burst into tears. I just didn't know how we were going to get through it. I couldn't ask Mum and Dad, and I knew my sisters were helping them out. We didn't have any answers. Mum rang to see how we were doing and I told her what had happened. They couldn't believe it.

I still didn't want to ask for help.

Thankfully my middle sister, Caroline, texted me and I ended up ringing her back. I told her I didn't know what to do. The very next day she flew up and stayed with us. She did all the cleaning and took care of the lawns; she picked the garlic, dug the potatoes, and took on lots of other jobs for us. She was brilliant.

In the meantime, we struggled to get Devon to the eye clinic and all the other places he needed to be, because he was in a wheelchair. He even had to sleep sitting up. He was on some pretty heavy drugs which made him hallucinate, and he couldn't go to work for a very long time. I still found what happened hard to believe, and I hated knowing that there was nothing I could personally do to fix it.

Throughout all of this I kept thinking I was going into labour, and then the feeling would stop. On and on it went, past the due date and into forty two weeks. Still no baby. And so they gave me a date of 21st January 2008 for an induction. Devon was going to come with me and Caroline planned to drive us there. But in the end, I had to ask Caroline to join us for the birth as my support partner, because unfortunately Devon was exhausted.

CHAPTER 4

THE BIGGEST BABY IN WAIRAU

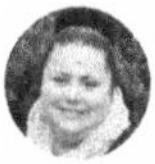

Sonya: Now, when I tell my story and I look back on everything that happened, it's hard to know how I coped with it all. Somehow, we just managed to keep going. I suppose we just didn't have a choice, or know any different at that stage.

I suppose I was living in a little bit of a dreamland. I didn't even stop to think about how I was going to manage to look after this baby with Devon being so unwell. He was still on tramadol and morphine and slept so much of the time, so he was a bit spaced out! And even though he wanted to be supportive, he struggled for obvious reasons.

On the morning of the induction, I was up early for the fifteen-minute drive to Wairau Hospital for my 7 am appointment. Devon and Caroline were both with me and I settled into Room 9, where I'd be staying for the next five or six days. Of course, I didn't know that at the time – I assumed I'd be having a normal vaginal birth and I'd be going home in a couple of days.

When they were ready to start the induction, they had to soften the cervix and get the ball rolling. They encouraged me to get up and go for a little walk, but things started to happen quite quickly ... I started to feel really sore, so that walk didn't last very long! I went from my hospital room into the birthing suite in the space of about two hours.

There was a clock in the birthing room and I remember thinking that wasn't such a great idea, because I ended up clock-watching and wishing the time would go faster. They pulled a big curtain around the bed but they left the door open beyond, so we could hear everything else that was going on. My midwife had a good talk with me about what to expect over the next few hours. It was pretty exciting.

They put the monitor on, and I could hear my little boy's heartbeat. It was nice and strong. The labour pains were starting to really kick in, and I asked for an epidural. It took about an hour for them to get the team down to come and put that into my back. It was pretty painful, but once it was in, it felt amazing. I couldn't feel anything, and yet the monitors definitely showed that my contractions were revving up. They were becoming increasingly regular, so it all seemed like the baby was going to come pretty quickly.

It was around midday and about 29 degrees, the hottest day of the year in Marlborough. It wasn't very nice at all. Caroline had ducked out to get souvlakia (Greek kebabs with grilled meat and vegetables) for Devon, herself and the midwife, which smelt absolutely amazing at the time (although the smell hung around after that!). I hadn't eaten since the night before, but they wouldn't let me eat anything in case I had to go in for an emergency caesarean section.

As the day progressed, my baby's movements and heart rate continued to look perfectly fine, and we were just going through the motions. But it was getting later and the hospital staff were changing shifts. The labour ward had been quite busy, so there had been a lady in the next room giving birth. She'd been quite loud, and that was scary.

A lot of people in my antenatal group were giving birth around about the same time – all at Wairau. So I had a couple of friends in there, but I didn't want to interfere in their family time.

It was starting to feel as if we were going to be in there forever at this stage. The obstetrician came down and examined me, but nothing seemed to be happening. I was still having the contractions, but my cervix wasn't dilating. They said the baby was quite big – but we didn't have any idea quite how big! And when they felt around baby's head, it appeared as if he was presenting as breech. In other words, he had twisted around so that he was lying with his feet first and his bottom facing down.

There was a real concern that I wouldn't be able to birth my baby naturally. I didn't feel ready to make that decision, but at around 8 pm we agreed that I should go for an emergency

C-section because things just weren't moving. After all the mental preparation, I suddenly had to accept the fact that I wasn't going to give birth naturally. I was going to be cut open so they could pull my baby out that way. He was going to be a sunroof baby, as they call it.

First, they had to break my waters, and that was an experience and a half. There was a sense of release like a balloon popping, and it was like I'd flooded the bed. I still couldn't actually feel my legs, but everything felt heavy.

Going into theatre was really scary. Devon and Caroline were all scrubbed up in their blues and came in with me. All I remember is being on the bed, going around lots and lots of corners, and looking at all the ceiling lights. My back felt sore and it seemed to take forever. We passed another lady who was holding a beautiful newborn baby girl, and I remember thinking, 'That's going to be me soon.' Looking back, I suppose the anticipation took its toll, but I didn't know any better. You just don't, the first time around.

We got to the theatre but the other obstetrician was still cleaning up. My own obstetrician took off for something to eat, so I wondered how long we were going to be there. In the meantime, the anaesthetist put some more epidural in and I was moved onto the bed.

And then, finally, it began ...

The midwife was there with Caroline standing next to her, and Devon was standing next to me. They asked if I wanted the sheet down, but I didn't think Devon would handle that very well, so I said we'd have the sheet up so we couldn't see. The anaesthetist was actually quite concerned as I'm allergic to an anaesthetic called cholinesterase. I'd had it once before when I had my tonsils out, but I'd been told that if I ever had it again, it would kill me. So the anaesthetist knew that if the C-section didn't go well, and they had to put me to sleep, they would have to be very careful about what drugs they used. I was really scared of the what-ifs: what if it did go wrong? What if I stopped breathing?

The next thing I remember was a whole lot of pulling and tugging. Someone said, 'It's going to feel like a rugby ball in there.'

Finally, at 9.10 pm on Monday 21st January 2008, Jack Roger Watson was born, weighing 10lb 14oz (4.9 kilos). He started crying pretty much immediately. He was very healthy and they scored him an eight and then a nine on the Apgar test, which assesses pulse, respiration, and all-round health after birth.

They cleaned him up, put him on the bed and the surgeons were looking at him apparently thinking, 'My goodness, how big is he?' Apparently, he was the biggest baby of all the babies born in Wairau in 2007. My midwife said there was no way he could have come out naturally!

Little did I know this was going to be a journey I hadn't prepared for. I hadn't read up about C-sections, I hadn't read up about healing. I didn't have a lot of information from antenatal class because that was all about vaginal deliveries. I had geared myself up for that, but that hadn't happened.

CHAPTER 5

'I LOOKED AT MY BABY, AND I FELT NOTHING'

Sonya: Once they'd checked he was all right they put Jack on my chest, but they very quickly took him away again to be suctioned as he was having a little difficulty breathing. When they brought him back they put him beside me, but not on me. I have a picture of Jack snuggled down into my arm, wrapped in a blanket, but there was no skin-to-skin contact at all. That was really difficult.

I looked at him and I didn't feel anything.

I should have been absolutely overjoyed. I knew I should be loving this baby, but there was absolutely no feeling there at all.

I couldn't believe it. I thought that these feelings would have just come to me naturally, straight after the birth. But they didn't.

When they took photos for the family album, I pretended to smile. I thought that was what everyone wanted to see.

We were wheeled into the recovery area. It was really dark, and I was the only new mother in there. There were two nurses in there talking about what time I was going to go back to my room on the maternity ward. The obstetrician had now gone home. But they didn't really talk to me and I just felt like I was in the way.

It had been just half an hour since I'd had my C-section. There was a drain coming out of my side, collecting blood. I had a catheter in, and there were some big puffy things going up and down on my legs to stop blood clots (given my father's history). I didn't know any of this was going to happen and I was mortified. They wheeled me back along the winding path to the maternity unit and all the wards were dark. It didn't feel very nice, and Jack was still lying there to the side of me.

Devon and Caroline were there waiting for us. The staff brought my placenta in to us in an ice cream container wrapped in a brown paper bag. My midwife came in and congratulated me. She told me the night nurses would look after me overnight and that she'd be back at eight in the morning to check on me and Jack. She suggested I try breastfeeding Jack, telling me she'd get the nurses to help me with that too.

Devon and Caroline were asked to leave the ward at around 11 pm. And when they left, I felt more alone that I'd ever felt in my life. Jack was back in his little crib. He was so big in it, he was actually touching the sides! He had a chubby, bright red face with a mop of dark hair like a little hedgehog. He gazed up at me. When he started to cry, I couldn't even get up to help him. I still couldn't move.

There were two midwives on duty that night, and they were like the Wicked Witches of the West! There were three of us from my antenatal group in there and we all had the same horrendous experience.

I rang my bell for help. One of the midwives came in, asking what I wanted. I told her my baby was crying and that I didn't know what to do. She told me she'd be back in a minute as she needed to get him started on breastfeeding. But that minute lasted a long time ...

Maybe twenty to thirty minutes later she came back in, and everything seemed like such an effort for her, as though helping me was a burden. It was a horrible experience. I didn't know what I was doing. She kept telling me to prop myself up and do this and do that – but he wouldn't even latch. He was crying and I was crying. I just wanted my husband and my midwife to be there with me.

We kept trying but nothing was working. I don't think anything even came out. Because I'd had a C-section, there was just no milk to come out. My breasts were getting more and more sore; it felt like the nurse was bruising me. After trying and failing for so long, she put Jack back in his crib. And I just lay there and watched the clock, counting down the hours till Devon arrived. I wanted to ring him and ask him to come in straightaway, but I knew I couldn't. We both had a really horrendous night.

I didn't get any pain relief that night. My drain was filling up quite quickly, and I was bleeding out of my vagina onto my bed.

I had to ring my bell again and ask them if they could help clean me up. One of them came back in and started to clean me, saying, 'What mess. Sonya, this is just a mess!' I told her I was sorry, and I felt like I needed to apologise for everything. But I was bleeding badly, and I couldn't help it.

The other midwives came in. One of them was a bit younger and a lot more reassuring, but then she got called away to a birth, so I ended up with the two wicked witches cleaning me up, talking among themselves. They asked me why I had blood on my hands, so I explained that I'd felt down there because it had felt like there was water running down my legs. So that set them off again: 'How are we going to wash your hands with you stuck on the bed?' They made out like everything was such an effort for them.

Part of me felt like getting up, taking my baby and walking out of there. But a bigger part of me couldn't even look at him.

They rolled me around a lot and cleaned the bed. If I could have, I would have done it myself. I didn't feel like that new mum I'd seen just a few hours before. I felt like just another number or statistic. By now my pain relief had worn off, but I wasn't given anything else.

At 6.30 am, I was asked to get up so they could take my drain and catheter out. I sat on the edge of the bed and they told me I might feel a bit dizzy. I did feel dizzy and I was in pain. But we still had to head off to the showers across the corridor, where I passed out on the floor. Apparently I'd passed out because I had no pain relief in my system, and it was just a few hours after I'd had a C-section. They'd given me absolutely nothing since I'd been in theatre.

The head midwife, the paediatrics (paeds) team and some of the charge midwives all came down and were pretty horrified to find me lying on the floor, unable to move. My C-section wound felt like it had buzzing bees inside it. I was in so much pain; it was the most awful feeling I have ever experienced.

With help, they got me up onto the bed and on some oxygen. The pain was so intense that they had to give me morphine. I was really looking forward to getting all the tubes out and getting cleaned up, but because the midwives hadn't given me the medication overnight, I wasn't allowed to shower. I was really disappointed, but I didn't complain about it.

The paeds team had been in to see Jack; he was quite jaundiced and had been getting worse overnight. He hadn't fed and he was very dehydrated. They decided to put him into phototherapy on a little bed with blue lights – it was a little bit like a mini sunbed, called a bili bed – that was supposed to help build up the colour in his skin. It was only supposed to be a short-term thing, but it lasted for three days. The first day he was there he didn't have a nappy on, and when he peed, the urine burnt his bottom.

He was in a little medical room that was filled with old chairs and equipment next to the main foyer. He was in there all by himself. I absolutely hated it. I couldn't stop thinking that someone was going to steal him – and if they did, I wouldn't even know. Who would hear him? He was miles away from my room. There wasn't even a nurse looking in on him. Here was this defenceless little baby lying all alone. I just wanted to hold him – or at least, to try to hold him and tell him it would all be okay.

Kathryn: Anxiety is an Important Feeling

Are you beginning to wonder how Sonya could have felt anything BUT anxiety at this point? Of course! Actually, the anxiety of being separated from her son and her fears about him being physically neglected were incredibly important emotions for Sonya to feel. Her anxiety was there to give her an important message: ACT NOW! Do something!

This is a great example of how cutting off, avoiding, and trying to get rid of our feelings can be incredibly unhelpful. Being present enough to listen to our feelings allows us to consider a vital question: 'Is this emotion a message about something important?' Being able to do this is no easy skill, but it can be so useful in these kinds of situations. Another way to do this is to connect with someone else and ask them to help you figure out the message your emotions are giving you, rather than the one your mind is trying to tell you.

No wonder Sonya developed fears her son might die: how could she not? They had both faced near-death situations.

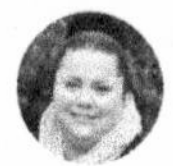

Sonya: When the paeds team brought Jack back in, they explained what had happened with the skin burn. He had burnt buttocks on both sides. They were absolutely mortified that it had happened, and me and Devon were too.

I didn't know what to do. I didn't want to ruffle feathers or get anyone into trouble. But, as a parent, I couldn't believe it. How do you burn a baby's bottom? How could anyone put him in there without a nappy on? There were so many unanswered questions.

And while all of that was happening, I was starting to go downhill. The baby blues were really kicking in. I was becoming more and more tearful. Just looking at myself in the mirror would cause me to cry. I tried to hide the tears that rolled down my face, but I couldn't stop them.

Poor Jack was on his own for three days, so I had three days of this agony. Staff would just bring him back to me to feed, but he still wasn't feeding properly. And so they had to feed him through a tube through his nose, but he kept trying to pull it out. Sometimes it would spill out and he'd scream loudly and continuously. The midwives would come in, ask what was wrong, and try to soothe him. I was desperate for their help.

I tried to express milk. The nurses used a breast machine, a big awful metal thing which they called Daisy! It looked like something from the 1920s. It was pretty scary-looking and they wheeled it in on a trolley. It was shared among everyone on the ward.

I tried to express, but it just wouldn't work. No milk came out and it seriously stressed me out. It wasn't until three or four days later that they said, 'Don't worry about it, you've had a C-section. Your body isn't ready, and your hormones aren't changing. Normally it would happen pretty much straightaway after a vaginal birth, but it could be up to a week after a C-section.' Why didn't they tell me that before?

I would often sit there crying at night, trying to pump milk using Daisy the pumping machine. The most I'd ever get at one time was fifteen ml of milk. It was so disappointing. I felt like a failure – I couldn't supply the one thing my baby needed.

With Jack coming in and out, it was hard to sleep. Whenever I tried, my mind would race and my anxiety would skyrocket. I couldn't stop worrying that someone would steal my baby. I don't think I ever even realised just how bad my anxiety about this was, until I started writing my story.

But the hardest thing – the thing that caused me the most anxiety – was knowing I didn't feel a bond with him. I didn't look at him and melt and think, 'Oh God, you're so beautiful.' There was nothing like that. On one level, I think I was just worried that if someone did take him, I wouldn't know how to explain it to everyone. And that was quite a strange feeling. I just didn't feel like I loved him.

Kathryn: An Incredible Mix of Feelings

I should explain more about this strange mix of feelings Sonya experienced here. I'm guessing this was possibly one of the most intense, emotional experiences she has ever experienced in her life. I think meeting your baby, and the first few days of life afterwards, often are. And surprisingly, when our emotions get that strong, sometimes all we can feel is numbness. Just think about the combination of things Sonya had to deal with:

- *Being starved and sleep-deprived for more than forty eight hours*
- *The massive physical achievement of labouring and the major C-section operation*
- *Her expectations of what her baby would be like and how she ought to feel at the time*
- *The flood of hormones that may or may not have been present*
- *The intensity of experiencing a close brush with life and death*

How could all of that NOT set any of us up for very weird emotional experiences? And there is even more to it than that.

Sonya's early experience with Jack is that she was numb and utterly overwhelmed. She had just had a massively traumatic experience: her life and her baby's life had been under threat. Human brains tend to move into survival mode in that kind of scenario. They become incredibly adaptive and can shut down feelings and emotions when huge amounts of potentially toxic adrenaline would otherwise flood the brain. This is a very normal response to trauma.

The awful part of this for Sonya and Jack was that it stopped Sonya from being able to connect immediately with him. Oxytocin (a hormone that's key to both bonding and lactation) is known as a shy hormone: it works best in intimate situations with dull lights and few people (certainly not strangers) around. Sonya's environment was opposite to that.

Instead, Sonya's fear system kicked in: she knew she needed to protect Jack. A similar effect would occur if Sonya's survival was threatened by a large predator, say a bear, immediately after giving birth. She would drop directly into survival mode and need to pick up Jack in order to run. If flight isn't an option, another survival strategy at that point is fighting or freezing. Either way, positive emotions are suppressed because they are unnecessary to survival in the short term. So I suspect Sonya's brain and body were doing what hundreds of thousands of years of evolution had so cleverly evolved them to do in order to survive. And this was devastating for her and Jack.

Then add into the equation all the death, threats of death, and threats to her physical wellbeing Sonya experienced in the lead up to the birth. There was her father's stroke, her friend's death from MS, Devon's major eye accident, topped by the C-section and the normal (and astounding) death threat that is birth. No wonder Sonya was preoccupied with Jack dying. And while that preoccupation continued, her mind was stuck in anxiety mode – re-living the trauma of the birth and obsessing about the importance of protecting her child.

Sonya: Once Jack came off the bili bed after three days, we tried bottle-feeding him – much to the midwives' disgust. But he didn't like that either, so he carried on being tube fed. The paediatrician diagnosed him with reflux on day three, so he started on medication for that pretty much straightaway.

Everything was hard. He had a loose larynx, so he sounded like an eighty-year old smoker when he breathed! It was all very gurgly. And the tube feeding was tough on him. Once he nearly choked on his food, and they had to resuscitate him. He actually turned purple. It was horrible.

Jack spent a lot of his time screaming. He almost screamed the place down at times. The midwives would take him and try to comfort him, but no one really knew what was wrong with him. I just wanted them to take him away. I didn't want to have to hear him anymore ... and I could hear him from down the hall. And all the time my anxiety continued to rise.

I thought about all the people I knew from the antenatal clinic, and I wondered what they were going to think. There they were with these babies that didn't scream and cry – and here was Jack, crying and crying non-stop. It was just bloody awful. I felt ashamed and embarrassed.

By this stage, my other sister Verity had come up to visit me and Caroline had gone back to Christchurch. Verity was driving Devon back and forth to the hospital, doing lunches and dinners and groceries. She was incredible. But I still really worried about Dev. I just wanted to be there to support him, and maybe that was why I felt the way I did with Jack. It wasn't a normal delivery, so I couldn't just go home to look after Dev as well.

So many things had gone wrong. The birth hadn't been anything like I'd imagined. I hadn't had any medication that first night. I couldn't breastfeed. Jack was on the bili bed for three days. Then there was the reflux diagnosis at three days old. (Little did we know that the reflux would last until he was three years old!) All the doctors told us he'd be over that within twelve weeks.

Being in that hospital didn't help either. It was tough not having my family around me, although I didn't feel like seeing people anyway. When someone did come and visit, I'd pretend to be asleep. I just didn't want to deal with anyone.

I felt like I was already failing at being a mother, and I hadn't even got home yet.

By day six in the hospital, I'd had more than I could take. I thought that Jack would be better off at home. I thought he'd stop crying once we got him out of there and home to his own little bassinet. I even thought that we could get him into some sort of routine. So I decided I would discharge myself. I know it sounds silly, but I went home for the night, and then ended up back in hospital the following night with severe pain through my C-section wound. I found out it was infected!

I was given pethidine and they put me back on a catheter. I was back on the maternity ward, but because I'd discharged myself early, they wouldn't do anything to look after Jack. So Devon had to come in and stay the night to look after him. I couldn't get off the bed to pick him up.

I really wish I'd put my hand up then and said, 'Look, I just can't do this.' Maybe things might have been different if I had. But I just battled on because I didn't know any better.

In the early hours of the next morning, Devon was down in the lounge, asleep. One of the midwives said to me, 'Oh, he's asleep. He needs his sleep.' Yet there I was, lying awake, thinking how much I needed sleep myself, but Jack was crying again. I was in such a huge room – it was the room for the mums who were on higher drug dosages – because they didn't have anywhere else to put me.

My C-section wound was sore and I just couldn't sleep. The buzzing bees were back, swarming around my stitch line. The obstetrician had come in and told me it was all fine. 'It's just in your head, Sonya!' she told me. 'So we'll be sending you home soon.'

It wasn't until they did the scan and the swabs came back that we realised just how badly it was infected.

CHAPTER 6

THE WORLD'S WORST MUM

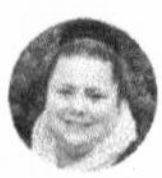

Sonya: After I saw the obstetrician and had the scan, they prescribed some pretty strong antibiotics and I was officially allowed to go home.

Being at home was obviously a lot better than being in hospital. But in truth, I really wanted to leave Jack behind, because I just didn't know what to do. Fortunately, we met a lovely lady who we called Nanny Barb, who was the receptionist in the maternity unit. I'd spoken to her, off and on, throughout my six days in hospital, and she was always so positive. She'd say things like, 'Sonya, you look great – and you've only just had a C-section!' She was so full of praise, and she'd often offer to take Jack for a walk around the ward for me.

Barb gave me her number – she must have felt sorry for me – and told me to call her if I needed any help. We found out that her husband was in the air force, so it was like our extended family reaching out to us again. Nanny Barb was just amazing. She rang to see how we were getting on the first night we were home.

That first night at home, we decided we were going to use paper plates for dinner. And we actually ended up doing that for the next few weeks. Devon didn't have the energy to clean up, I could hardly walk, and life with Jack was pretty demanding. He hardly stopped crying or vomiting.

On the third night, we were sitting on a couch in Jack's room and Devon and I looked at each other. It was as if the thought had passed between us: *What the fuck have we done?*

Having this baby – this whole experience – was so totally different from what we'd expected. Jack just cried constantly. I was so worried that everyone would hear him and think I couldn't handle the baby. I knew that Devon was exhausted, and I was exhausted. I just wanted someone to take my baby away from me.

We needed help. Mum and Dad had called, and Mum was trying to arrange to come and see us, but she still needed to look after Dad. And then Devon's parents called to congratulate us. But no one was around. It was as if everyone had disappeared and we were on our own, trying to cope with this baby.

We ended up having trips in and out of hospital, and one night in particular Jack just wouldn't stop screaming. I had got to the point where I no longer knew what to do with him. And so he was admitted to paediatrics.

There were a couple of awesome doctors on that night who took a bit of a liking to Jack. One of them told us that his son had had severe reflux, so he knew what we were going through. He tried to settle Jack for over an hour, but he just kept on crying. We tried a dummy, we tried bottle-feeding with a choo-choo teat, but nothing was working. They took blood and urine samples, and Devon ended up staying with him that night.

I went home alone – and it was a strange feeling. There was a lot of guilt. I felt like the world's worst mum.

Kathryn: *I feel such compassion for Sonya going through all of that. How painful to have such an awful experience when you're anticipating a joyful start to your family. First you have that idea stolen away from you, and then, on top of that, you come to believe that everything that's gone wrong is your fault.*

Deciding she was "the world's worst mum" so early on reflects the horrible sense of loneliness that Sonya and Devon were feeling. Sonya was stoic and set huge expectations for herself. I wish I could go back there and tell Sonya she was doing the best that she could. After all, that's the most we can ever do. And I would especially like to tell her, 'It's not your fault. You are not to blame. Nor must you be alone in this.'

I would be very surprised if most mothers in our culture don't think they're the world's worst mum at some point. Imagine for a moment this army of mothers, this massive group of people who have taken on so much guilt. Can they all be so awful? Do they all deserve such harsh judgement? Remember that you are one of them.

See if you can let go – just a little – of the judgement you hold against yourself. Apply a little of the compassion you might be experiencing towards Sonya to your own experience as a mother. Even if, right now, you think that your experience was nowhere near as bad as Sonya's, see if you can still show yourself some of that compassion. It's why Sonya is sharing her story with you: you are not alone.

Sonya: These feelings of guilt resurfaced a lot over the next few weeks. At one stage the hospital staff looked at us, and said, 'Look, leave him here. We've got no one else on the ward. We'll look after him for the night.' So, at 1 am, Devon and I walked out of that hospital together. It was a warm summer evening in Marlborough, and I felt such huge relief. I felt like leaving Jack in there and never going back. I just wanted *so much sleep!*

We got home and I saw Jack's bassinet in his room. I wanted to be able to just tuck it away and leave him at the hospital for the next month. They could take care of him. But then the guilt hit me again, and it was awful. I was upset that I felt this way, but I just didn't want him to come home.

We managed to get some sleep, but everything was quickly back to normal the next morning when we picked Jack up. The guilt struck me again when we arrived at the hospital. It felt like everyone was watching us when we walked in. It felt like they were thinking, *Look, it's those parents who dropped their baby off for the night!*

And I could hear Jack! He was crying and the nurses were trying to calm him, but it wasn't working.

We had another meeting with the paeds team. Jack's samples had come back positive with a urinary tract infection. So here's this baby with a UTI, on antibiotics, at just eight or nine days old. And I blamed myself. Was it the way we had cleaned his penis that had given him a UTI? The sense of self-blame was huge.

I couldn't understand how it could happen – how does a baby get a urinary tract infection? The doctors didn't know either. That was just the start of a long string of UTIs for Jack, and nobody really knew why he developed them. The first time they scanned him, nothing showed up – his kidneys looked fine. So they put him on a prophylactic antibiotic which he had to take every day. At nine days old, he was taking ranitidine, domperidone, and Gaviscon – we had to keep a notebook of all the medication he was receiving. I felt even worse having to give my little baby all this medicine. I was so ashamed, I couldn't even tell anyone.

Those feelings of guilt – and all the questions about why my child needed this medicine – were getting harder to deal with. We knew what they were for, but no one really explained what was going on. We didn't know how long he'd have to take it all, or what the long-term effects were going to be. There was not a lot of support.

Devon went back to work in February 2008, at about week three. The older ladies at work told him that Jack just needed feeding up. They said he was just hungry and that's why he was crying. So they were sending Devon home with baby food, for goodness' sake! I was mixing up this stuff and spoon-feeding this little baby who was only a few weeks old. It was ridiculous, but I didn't know any better.

Then there was colic powder, and reflux powder, and all sorts of other suggestions – all these people knew what was wrong with my baby. So why didn't I know what they knew? That really wasn't a nice feeling.

I ended up throwing most of the baby food out. It was some kind of white powder. Who knew what was in it? Not that I thought anyone was trying to do him any harm, but we were already giving him so much medication anyway. And anyway, nothing seemed to be working. This child just screamed. He wouldn't settle. He vomited up most of his feeds but continued to put weight on and we couldn't work out why.

Devon and I had got to the stage where we were just going through the motions. My infection was still healing and I still wasn't meant to be driving, so it was hard with Devon being back at work. He was only working half-days to begin with because he was still so physically and mentally exhausted. It was nice having him come home early, but it was still hard because he would just go straight to bed and I still had to deal with this crying baby.

My midwife would still come and visit, but they were down to weekly visits now. She weighed him each time, and every time his weight kept on going up. He was still on the prophylactic antibiotic – and that would last for seven or eight months. He was still on all the other meds too, so he still needed to be checked by the paeds team every couple of weeks. There was still some concern that even though he was so big, he still had a loose larynx, the reflux, and lots of other little things going on that nobody had any answers for.

Every time in paeds, we'd bump into Nanny Barb. One day she offered to take Jack for a night, and I couldn't believe it. At the time, I didn't know if they secretly questioned whether they thought Jack was really crying or whether I was making it up. But when she offered, I was so grateful. We dropped him off round at her place and although it was a bit of a strange feeling – to be dropping our baby off at somebody else's house – I didn't really care. It was just so nice to have a night off.

It sounds so terrible when I say that, but I just needed someone to take him.

Sure enough, the next morning we found out that they'd had a pretty awful night with him. He had been crying most of the time and had just napped in small segments. He'd also vomited up his milk. Nanny Barb simply said, 'I don't know how you're doing it.' It was the first time anyone had really acknowledged how hard it was for us.

'I'm not coping,' I told her. 'This is really hard. Is this normal – is this a normal baby?'

She said, 'Well, normal babies cry, but normal babies don't scream. They don't vomit up their milk every feed ... I feel for you.'

Nany Barb told me she was going to tell the paeds team what was happening. So maybe they had spoken to her, I don't know. I don't think they believed me when I said he didn't sleep at all, no matter what we did. We'd have him in the pram going over bumps in the road, or on the lino inside, and he still wouldn't sleep. We'd put him in his capsule car seat and he wouldn't sleep. We even hired a baby swing with a half capsule in it and it was supposed to swing *any* baby to sleep. It didn't swing Jack to sleep. He just vomited!

We tried everything. Absolutely everything. But no matter what we tried, he just would not settle. So paeds switched to weekly checks because things obviously weren't improving. There were still so many questions that weren't being answered.

Were we doing things wrong as parents? I was trying to read all the books and magazine articles I could find to get as much information as I could. I felt like we needed to educate ourselves more because it really did look like we didn't know what we were doing as parents. I really struggled with that sense of not being able to work it out – I'd thought it was going to be a lot easier than everything we'd experienced so far.

Mum and Dad were pretty concerned, and they felt bad because it was so hard for them to visit. In the end, Mum did manage to come up and she couldn't believe what Jack was like. So it was really nice for us to have someone else in the house to help with meals. We weren't even eating properly; we were still eating on paper plates! So it was really good to have her there.

Then Devon's parents did a surprise trip and turned up with everyone in tow. They expected us to put a meal on for them, and I was in no space to be able to do that. Very diplomatically, Devon suggested we'd do a barbeque, but it'd help if they brought their own meat and drink. Thank goodness my mum was there because she did all the salads and got everything ready.

It was really hard. Everyone sat round with this crying baby, and Dev's mum took him and said, 'There, there, Jack. I'll stop you crying ...' She couldn't! Secretly I was laughing because it felt good to have physical proof that I wasn't lying. I was being made out to be a failure in my job as a mum and a wife. I'd been made to feel that way as soon as they'd walked through the door. Dev's dad walked in and gave me the biggest hug and congratulated us, but his mum just walked right past me.

I expected to have a mother- and father-in-law who would be amazing and supportive, who would want to take Jack and hold him. But it wasn't like that at all. They left after the barbeque, but they wanted to come around the next day for morning tea. There were a lot of expectations about what we should have been doing to host them, but nothing in the way of help. We could have really used a hand mowing the lawn, for example. And then there were some jealous questions about why my mum was staying with us, even though she was doing all this work to try to support us.

In the end we gave in to them and we did morning tea ... and afternoon tea. We did the dutiful host bit. Then they went to the coast for a few days, and my mum stayed on to help.

A few days later we got a phone call. Surprise! They were back in Bleiheim. And they expected lunch!

'No, enough's enough,' I said. 'I can't do it.'

But they turned up anyway, and Dev's mum got really angry. Devon was sitting in Jack's room and she came storming in, demanding to know why we didn't want to see them. So Devon explained it to her. It was all a bit scary, so I was hiding in our bedroom. I was just too tired to deal with it. I knew I was at meltdown stage too.

Dev's mum was screaming at him, 'Why won't you let us stay? What have we done?'

Devon simply said, 'For fuck's sake, get out of my house!'

And that was that. Since he was just a few weeks old, Jack has not seen his grandparents. He has never been acknowledged by them again.

We spent the best part of a year sending letters and photos, but got nothing back. Devon still made a point of contacting them every month to tell them what was happening. And every month, the call would end with them hanging up on him. Sometimes his mum would get angry and abuse Devon or abuse me. She called me a wet fish. She never showed me any empathy.

She always seemed like such a controlling lady. And it just went on until the stage where we'd had all we could take. I couldn't believe someone's parents could be like that. I couldn't believe they didn't want to be a part of Jack's life.

It was a huge learning curve for us. It's taken a long time to even accept it – although in a way, I still don't. I don't understand how someone could be like that, how they could switch off a family member like that, especially their own grandchild! They don't show any interest in their grandson, the boy who carries the Watson name ... it did even make us question whether we should change Jack's last name. I know Devon has accepted it, but still he struggles with the fact that his own parents won't even talk to him.

CHAPTER 7

PRETENDING EVERYTHING WAS OKAY

Sonya: At around the time Jack was three months old, he had another scan on his kidney. They found that he had kidney stones. So this explained the ongoing urinary tract infections. It also helped explain why he was crying all the time – if it wasn't because of the reflux, it was because of the pain of the kidney stones.

He carried on taking the prophylactic antibiotic and we continued the many, many visits to our doctor and Wairau Hospital. All this time, Jack continued to grow. He was getting quite a bit bigger and moved out of his bassinet into a cot at just three weeks old. None of the beautiful newborn clothes fit him anymore and we were already up to the next nappy size. But still he kept on growing. He didn't feel like a little snuggly baby; he was just so big.

He was still crying lots and I was really beginning to hate what we had created.

I know that is such a strong word to use, but at that time I felt like I would do anything to go back to my life before I had a baby. Life back then was so easy – and so stress-free.

Life with Jack was really hard. I didn't expect that we would be going back and forth to hospitals and doctors and worrying about him all the time. I never imagined I wouldn't have had a bond with him. And because of all the medical issues, I didn't even feel like I'd birthed a baby.

The days rolled into each other. We managed to get some funding through Plunket, the health visiting service, and they sent out a lovely Karitane nurse – that's a nurse specially trained to work with babies. She helped me out two or three times a week. She used to take Jack for a walk around the airfield which was just a few blocks away, and still he would cry and cry. She didn't know what to do with him either.

I would often try to have a quick sleep in the bedroom, but I felt so worried thinking about whether or not she'd managed to stop him crying. And then I'd hear her coming back down the road with Jack still crying away, non-stop.

Nevertheless, I really looked forward to those one or two hours of freedom. It meant that I could do simple things like go out and get the groceries without taking a screaming baby. It was an incredible feeling to get out on my own. I didn't want to go home! I didn't want to have to deal with Jack when I got back to reality.

Devon was getting better slowly, but he still often felt exhausted. And he was still suffering the aftereffects of what had happened with his parents. Because things were still so difficult, we made the decision that Devon should ask for a transfer to Christchurch. He spoke to his bosses about his health, as well as Jack's and my own. My C-section was still open at one end, and I was taking antibiotics on and off. When I went back to the obstetrician and told her it felt like there were bees stinging me all along the stitch line, she kept implying it was all in my head – although she was careful not to say that exactly.

The air force was amazing. They sorted out a transfer for us and they packed up our house. I had such mixed feelings: I loved the memories we had made in that wee house, but I knew we had to move. I couldn't cope.

We were transferred out to Burnham army camp, about half an hour outside of Christchurch. I was so excited to move there, imagining how amazing it was going to be to have all that family support. I thought everything was going to be so easy ... but little did we know it was going to be terrible.

The house was disgusting. It obviously hadn't been cleaned for a very long time. There was dog poo all over the back section, and the low fences looked out over everyone else's houses. There was no privacy. I felt like a goldfish in a bowl. It was especially awful knowing what we'd given up, but I knew I had to be grateful. We had managed to get to Christchurch. Dev was working out of Wellington now and had to make quite a few trips there and back every week. In hindsight, that wasn't so great. But we were closer to Christchurch – and my family – and we felt that Jack would get better health support there.

But it didn't pan out the way I expected.

I really felt the isolation of living out in Burnham. I could feel my depression getting worse, and that's when I really knew that things were starting to spiral. I got to the point where I didn't want to have a shower when I got up in the morning. I didn't even want to go outside. Dev would ask me why I didn't go for a walk around the base, but I couldn't think of anything worse. I couldn't believe he'd even suggested it. I couldn't even get dressed.

I would find any excuse not to go walking – any excuse at all. Some days I would just sit on the couch and not move. I felt like I was stuck. I knew I just had to get through the basics of dealing with Jack, and I really struggled with that. I struggled even more living in a damp house as we moved towards our first winter in Burnham. There were mice in the house. There was no dry wood to make a fire. It was all so ramshackle.

Sometimes I'd look out on all my neighbours' houses. The neighbourhood was so different from Woodbourne where we'd looked out onto a beautiful vineyard and rolling hills. We didn't have a vegetable garden anymore. The gardens were a mess.

I know all these things seem so minor when I look back at them, but they really fuelled my postnatal depression, along with the lack of sleep, the screaming baby, and all the regular hospital check-ups on Jack's kidney stones.

I started to get anxious about Devon leaving too. Two days before he'd be due to fly out, my anxiety would start to build. What would I do if the plane crashed? How would I manage? I'd be stuck with this baby and I wouldn't know how to sort him out on my own.

Whenever Devon was in Wellington, and I was stuck in Burnham with the baby without any friends, I felt isolated. I didn't know anyone there.

It didn't help that Devon was in the air force, and we were on an army base. There seemed to be a definite separation. There was a family wellbeing lady on the base, and she'd come around sometimes, but she didn't actually offer me any support. She suggested we go to a playgroup, and I tried to go. I did all the things you're supposed to do – I fed Jack and tried to get him to sleep before we went, because I was so worried about what people would think. I knew I had to give it a try.

But then, when I got to the playgroup, I walked just right past instead. I just couldn't go in. I saw all the mums getting out of their cars and they looked happy. And their toddlers all looked happy in their little jackets and gumboots.

They were all so happy – what would they do when Jack started crying and screaming and vomiting? What would I tell them when they wanted to know why he cried? Or why he was so unsettled? Or why he vomited up his food? I wasn't even breastfeeding – what would they think of me for that?

I was scared of their judgement.

I really struggled with it because I really wanted to be able to join in. I'm quite a sociable person, so I wanted – *I needed* – to be a part of these groups. It was one of the things I'd looked forward to about becoming a mum.

Of course, if I'd known what I know now, I would have said, 'Bugger it, I'm going! And I don't bloody care who says what!' But the first time around, it's not like that. It's so hard, whether you have a healthy baby or a sick baby. Parenting is bloody hard work.

It doesn't matter what other people think; it's your baby, and what they think doesn't actually matter. I wish someone had told me that sooner! If they had, I might have seen things a bit differently.

But back then, my depression was pretty raw and it was getting worse. I was struggling, but I just put on my mask and pretended it was okay. I was seeing a new Plunket lady in Burnham, and she suggested we should put Jack into pre-school for a couple of half-days every week.

Devon came with me when I signed Jack up, and I was in tears. The guilt was overwhelming. I wasn't going to work; I was putting my six-month old child into day care so that I could have a break. Who sends their child to pre-school at that age when they're not working? That's not the right thing to do, is it?

And what did I do on my half-days off? I cleaned! I obsessed about cleaning, tidying, and gardening. I was supposed to spend the time catching up on my sleep, but I never did.

On the days I'd drive down and drop him off, I would sometimes think, *What if I didn't pick him up? What if I just left him there?*

I felt like a huge failure, like I was letting our child down. And yet, they loved him at pre-school. He thrived there. They would show me all these pictures of him sitting in the sandpit or in the baby area, looking content. And I would think, *Why can't I do that?*

Now, I have photos of my children everywhere – but back then there were hardly any of Jack as a baby. And that still makes me sad.

CHAPTER 8

THE HURRICANE WAS BUILDING

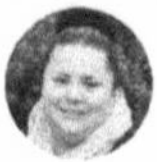

Sonya: My mental health continued to go downhill. The cleaning was becoming more obsessive. I felt the expectation of having a scrupulously clean and tidy house because I was at home all the time. I was still fixating on the thought of Devon's plane crashing and trying to cope with all the anxiety and worry around that.

When Dev was away, my sisters would come and stay with me in the evenings and bring a meal with them. Mum came out a few times too.

As well as the anxiety, I was really starting to feel a lot of anger. Mostly this was about why Jack wasn't a normal baby. Why couldn't I have had a baby who slept or breastfed normally?

We were getting help and support from the paeds team, but nothing seemed to change. Jack just kept on crying. There were only very short moments of time when he wasn't crying. And because he only slept in little bursts, it meant it was very difficult for us to get any sleep. My sleep patterns were terrible. Jack was waking every hour - and I know that's quite normal for a young baby. But by this point he was six months old, and a baby of that age should be able to sleep a little bit longer.

I became more and more sleep deprived, and I have always been a person who really needs their sleep. I can sleep sitting up, I can sleep in a chair, I can sleep anywhere! So the sleep deprivation was crippling, and it was making me more and more angry. Why couldn't I just have a baby who slept? Every night, we made sure he was changed, he was warm, and he was fed ... but I think that by now, he was starting to pick up on my feelings too. Was that contributing to him not settling and not sleeping properly?

My fuse was now very, very short! Of course, I wouldn't hit Jack or hurt him in any way, but I would feel the anger creeping up inside of me, like a hurricane starting to twirl.

During the day I would walk around like a zombie, my brain in a fog. I struggled to remember what I was meant to be doing day by day. I could cope with the basics, but I had to write appointments down. My memory had always been so good, but now I had to make lists so I could remember what to buy at the supermarket. It was all so frustrating. I felt as if I was grieving, in a sense. As if I had lost so much of myself.

I still didn't want to leave the house in case someone saw me or heard Jack crying. Even going out to the clothesline felt difficult. Because of the low chicken-wire fences, I felt as if everyone could see me, so I couldn't just pop out in my pyjamas. I was still so worried about what other people would see and hear and think.

A crying baby is a bit like a crying dog, but worse. You feel like people are asking themselves, *What's wrong with that baby? Why won't he stop crying?* I worried about it all the time.

But now, you know what I'd think? I'd think, *Who cares?* If I hear a crying baby, I don't think *What's wrong with that baby, why won't it shut up?* I think, *That poor mum!*

It wasn't just the mental stress that was causing me issues. My stitch line still hadn't healed properly and I was getting constant headaches. My body ached, my feet were sore, and I ended up with ingrowing toenails which I needed surgery on. I don't remember ever not aching during that time, and I think that was another symptom of the depression.

I was waking up with headaches. I wasn't drinking enough water, and I wasn't eating properly. I just didn't have the motivation to eat. I would skip meals and then wonder why I felt so faint! Devon would leave little snacks of nuts, fruit, and crackers for me because it was just too hard for me to go to the fruit bowl and get myself a piece of fruit. My motivation to do anything was gone, except for cleaning. I couldn't look after myself, but at least the house was absolutely spotless!

Further down the line I learnt just how important self-care is. I already knew that, of course, but it all went down the drain after I had Jack. It got to the point where Devon would have to take me to the shower before he went to work. I couldn't even be bothered to get undressed. I didn't have any motivation to go and buy new clothes; I just wanted to stay inside and do nothing. I didn't have any hobbies. I had nothing else in my life.

I felt like I lost myself.

I had no sexual interest. I remember thinking that it wouldn't bother me if I never had sex again for the rest of my life. And that's terrible. I know that, after having a baby, your sexual interest reduces, but just the thought of it was awful. I felt as if I wanted a bubble around me so no one could touch me. I ached too much. I would ache if someone touched my hand or touched my shoulder. I couldn't think of anything worse than sexual intercourse.

I was in a marriage, and having those desires and needs is a part of marriage. But I just wanted to shut everyone out, even Devon. I wouldn't make phone calls; I wouldn't even answer the phone. Devon had to make all the phone calls to arrange appointments.

The only person I would speak to on the phone was Devon. I couldn't even speak to my family, so he had to fill them in on everything that was happening. I don't think they really understood what was going on with me. They would only have known what I told Devon. If they read this, it will be the first time that people will get a real sense of what was going on in my head. At the time, I just didn't want anyone to know.

All my family really knew was that I was struggling with Jack. They wouldn't have known about the anger, the lack of motivation, the aches and the anxiety. I put the happy mask back on and hid as much as I could. And if anyone asked me how I was doing, I'd tell them I was fine. It was easy to put the mask on – why would you want to bother people with all your problems? Everyone has problems. Why would I want to drop all of mine on someone else?

The hurricane was building, with lots of things going round and round in my head. And that's when I started to think: *What if I wasn't here? What if I just died?*

I only had a few of those thoughts, but one in particular really stood out. I was driving back from the hospital with Jack and he was crying and crying. And just for a second, I thought, *What if I just drive into a tree or a lamppost? It'd all be over. I wouldn't have to deal with all the thoughts, or the pain, or the confusion anymore.*

This isn't what being a mother is supposed to be like. This isn't what the glossy magazine show. They show happy mothers – with happy babies breastfeeding beautifully. Babies who go to sleep straightaway. They show women who are happy with their baby and happy in their marriage. I wasn't that person.

The magazines make parenting look so amazing. They told me it was going to be a beautiful experience. But it sucked. I didn't have any of the things they promised. I hated Burnham, and I hated how I was feeling. I struggled with my baby every hour of every day. And I struggled with how it had changed my life and my marriage.

Devon and I were still in love though, and through it all Devon was bloody amazing! He just stuck in there. He did everything he could to help me. He cooked and came home early to work from home so he could be with me.

I wasn't very grateful at that time. I know I put a lot of guilt on him. I was tired of feeling the anxiety every time he got on a plane. *Has it landed safely? Is he all right? Will he find someone else – someone who can make him happier?* I was so insecure. I just wanted him to be there for me. I felt like my life had crashed.

Motherhood wasn't like I'd expected at all. I thought I would be so happy that we'd had a boy, happy that we were near Christchurch, and happy to join all these happy playgroups. But I wasn't. Not at all.

I saw a doctor and told them about my feelings. They got the gist of it. I was told I had postnatal depression and was sent away with Prozac. But I hadn't even really told them everything that was going on. I was too worried that Jack was going to be taken off me ... and how bad would that look? I couldn't tell them I had no bond with my baby either, so I kept it to myself.

The doctor referred me to the Postnatal Adjustment Programme (PNAP) in the Canterbury region of New Zealand. But that came with a seven-week waiting list. I thought I'd be dead by then. It just felt like no one wanted to know.

CHAPTER 9

'POSTNATAL DEPRESSION? HERE'S A WEBSITE, GO AND LOOK AT IT'

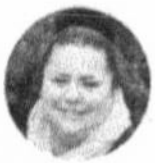

Sonya: By the time Jack was seven months old, Plunket was becoming a lot more involved in his life. We normally saw a lady called Chris, but one time we saw an older lady and it felt to me like she didn't really enjoy her job. She was very cold.

She sat down and took a couple of calls on her phone, then asked about Jack. I showed her his Plunket health book, which runs from birth to five years old. It records all his health and weight checks, his sight, hearing, speech, language, learning, and behaviour milestones. There are spaces to record where your child is at with rolling, crawling and (in time) taking their first steps. Jack already had quite a long list of appointments and information in his book!

This lady hadn't read Jack's notes, so I had to fill her in on the reflux, the kidney stones, and everything else. She asked if I'd tried breastfeeding, and I told her it hadn't worked. But she wanted to know why it hadn't worked, which made me feel very judged.

I told her how he was on three different types of medication under paediatric advice, but she made out that he couldn't possibly be as bad as they'd made him out to be, saying that he was a "good, strong lad". Jack was certainly growing. His head was big and he was long. His weight was in the 97th percentile for his age. He was already on solids. And that made me think that maybe she was right. Maybe he wasn't that unwell after all, and maybe he shouldn't have been in and out of hospital. He wasn't even crying when she was there.

What we didn't know at the time was that Jack had Sotos syndrome. It's a genetic disorder that can start in the womb – which explained why Jack was such a big baby – that leads to abnormal growth. It can be accompanied by delayed development in motor skills, poor muscle tone, and speech impairment, among others.

If we'd known about Sotos back then, it would have answered a lot of questions about why he continued to grow so big so quickly. It helped explain the health issues too – they were all part of Sotos. But the tell-tale signs – the big forehead and the slanted eyes – weren't really visible in Jack. And it was rare. Even our local doctor hadn't heard of it, so no one really picked up on the possibility.

The visit did not go well. After she'd answered her phone a few more times, I built up the courage to tell her that I thought I had postnatal depression. She said, 'Here's a website, go and look at it.' But that was all she did. She didn't talk to me about it at all. And so again I wondered if maybe, just maybe, the doctors had got it wrong.

Depression was such a scary word. As I write, we're only looking back eight years, but even then it wasn't talked about as much as it is now. I related it to the old Sunnyside mental hospital that I remembered from my childhood in Christchurch – and that was a scary thought.

It felt like there was such a stigma attached to the word, unfortunately. And I really didn't like that label: postnatal depression. But there are no two ways about it – that is bloody well what I had! But this lady didn't want to know.

Devon was away that week, and I suppose that I was reaching out to the Plunket lady for something ... maybe it was her support I needed. Or maybe I was just looking for someone to say, 'Hey, it's okay.' But she didn't give me that, and after she left, I felt so empty. I just cried and cried, and then Jack started crying. The memory of that visit is still so raw even now. She just didn't get it. She was supposed to be there for the mother and the baby, but she didn't want to know about me. And I think that's really sad. We lived in such an isolated area, and I can't help wondering just how many other mums were being ignored.

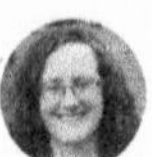

Kathryn: Not Being Heard and Not Being Held

Tragically, as Sonya intimates, this experience of being met with coldness when a mother discloses her PND is far from unusual. If this has been your experience, it's not good enough. And the hard part is that new mothers are not often in a position of sufficient power or confidence to either ask for what they need or give health professionals feedback about this kind of reaction.

If this is the case for you, we give you full permission to seek out what you need. It is okay to ask to change workers. It is okay to keep saying you need help until you find someone who can give you the care you need. And if you cannot speak for yourself, or you're tired of battling to be heard, tell someone else and ask them to help you find someone who will speak on your behalf. You deserve this, your baby deserves it, and your family deserves it.

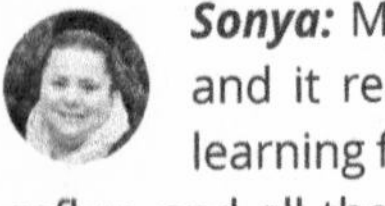

Sonya: My usual Plunket nurse, Chris, was so amazing, and it really felt like she was on the journey with us, learning from Jack's experiences – the kidney stones, the reflux, and all the scans. It was almost like a learning curve for her too. She was a beautiful person. I just wanted to take her home so she could look after us! I think I even said she could take Jack and look after him – and then of course, I laughed it off.

Those two were some of the people I remember most vividly from our journey. And there were so many other people who came in and out of our story. I remember all the people who'd say, 'What a big, bonny baby!' and then I'd tell them he was only eight months old and they couldn't believe it. They'd think he was twice that age and they'd want to know why he wasn't rolling or crawling yet!

Because of the Sotos syndrome, Jack's bones grew faster than his muscles did. As a result, he wasn't going to be able to hit any of his milestones. But of course, no one told me that. You have all these expectations as a parent. You read books and magazines, and Google tells you that your child should be doing this or that – but I didn't know about the Sotos syndrome. So I blamed myself for every missed milestone. I wondered if it was because we weren't going to playgroup, but really it was just a symptom of the syndrome.

Chris had recommended I try a reflux group in Rolleston, and I met another mum with a baby who just cried all the time. That was the first time I had seen another baby that I could compare with Jack. The mum talked about how hard it was for her and her husband to sleep at night, and of course I knew exactly what she was going through.

That was a bit of an eye-opener. It felt, for the first time, as if I wasn't the only one with such an unsettled baby.

The next few months were just as full of appointments, and there were a couple of hospital admissions too when Jack was particularly unsettled. One time in particular, when Devon was away, I went in with Jack because I just couldn't settle him. He was screaming and screaming, so I drove him thirty-five miles to the Accident and Emergency department at Christchurch Public Hospital. Because we got there so early we were able to park right outside the entrance – and over time it became a bit of a family joke. That was Jack's parking space!

Jack was screaming the place down, so they took him straight in. There was an older lady doctor on duty, and she'd seen a bit of his history. She said it was probably just the kidney stone releasing itself, and they decided to keep an eye on him.

That meant we had to wait in A&E. He wasn't in a cot or anything; we were just sitting on a slimline hospital bed in the middle of A&E. I had no one to hold him. I wasn't allowed to feed him – just in case they needed to take him in for surgery. I just tried to keep him occupied with his dummy. A&E was getting busier and busier and everyone was looking over at us because I couldn't keep him quiet.

I felt so alone. Jack just carried on screaming the place down. The doctor had given him some painkiller as his temperature was a bit high. But that didn't have any effect, so she gave him another lot and he slowly settled down. They thought the kidney stone was going to pass and considered taking him into surgery, so Dev got a flight home. It made me feel really guilty that I couldn't handle things on my own, but he came straight to the hospital to give me a break from holding Jack.

We sat in A&E for most of the day. The paeds team came and looked at him and took some urine samples. Once again he had another UTI, and that was probably why he was in so much pain. It was burning him so much when he peed.

The kidney stone still wasn't ready to pass, so they sent us home.

That was our life. It was one ordeal after another. They put Jack on antibiotics, but they were stronger than he was used to and brought him out in a rash. So then they had to try different antibiotics to try to clear this UTI.

I was constantly giving him medication and it felt like I was poisoning my baby. How many babies do you know who are on so much medication? That just made me feel even more guilty – I couldn't give my son a good life. The poor little bugger was in and out of hospital all the time. It was always one appointment after another. His first year of life was horrendous.

CHAPTER 10

'THEY TOLD ME MY LITTLE BOY WAS GOING TO DIE'

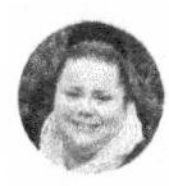

Sonya: It was getting harder and harder to put my happy mask on every day. I cried a lot. I would cry in the shower (if I could be bothered to get in the shower). I cried whenever Devon wasn't there. Most of the time I just wanted to go to bed and sleep, but I couldn't. I had to be there for Jack.

It was difficult: even though I felt angry with Jack, even though we had no bond and I felt like I didn't love him, I knew I had to be there for him. That was my responsibility as a parent.

I still found it hard to talk to friends. I couldn't talk to Mum and Dad because I didn't want them to be stressed out. I didn't even want them to know what was going on. And we still didn't have any contact with Dev's parents, despite all of his efforts. We didn't have that support that I'd always thought we'd have.

It wasn't until I went back to the doctor that my mask finally slipped. I saw a really lovely doctor, and it was absolutely okay that I cried in front of her. She said that what was happening to me wasn't good enough and referred me to the mothers and babies unit at Christchurch Hospital (for mums with severe postnatal depression). It was so good thinking that someone there might listen to me and actually understand what I was going through.

My medication was also increased but I struggled to take it. More than that, I think I struggled to accept that I was so unwell, or that I needed so much help. But things were going downhill fast; this time, I really did need help.

At home, Devon was moving heaven and earth to help me. He already had an amazing bond with Jack, and of course I couldn't help but be jealous of that. Jack was the apple of his eye. I was the one who had carried Jack, and yet it was Devon who had that amazing bond, not me. I struggled with that. I didn't know if I would ever have a bond with my son. And so, for all those months, I just had to pretend. I was pretty good at hiding things after all.

There are a lot of things I wish I'd known before I had Jack. They only devoted a singular ten-minute talk to mental health issues at antenatal class, and no one ever said, 'It's okay to have antenatal or postnatal depression. It's okay to feel anxious when your baby cries. It's okay to ask for help.'

When you don't think it's okay, you just feel like the world's biggest failure as a mum for not wanting this baby or for wanting your life to go back to what it was. But I did want my old life back, and I know how sad that sounds.

There was a long waiting list for the referral, so I continued seeking support from my doctor and PNAP. Shelley was incredible. She was like my guardian angel. I tried to go to a couple of the PNAP Cognitive Behavioural Therapy groups, but I really struggled, so I made up every excuse under the sun not go to. A couple of times I made the forty-five-minute drive with the intention of going, but I couldn't even go in. There were times when I didn't even really know how I'd got there, I was so sleep deprived. I'd been running on empty for so long, I would have quite happily slept forever. But life went on ...

Every day felt the same. I was just going through the motions. By ten in the morning, I'd be counting down the hours until Dev got home. And if anyone knocked at the door during the day, I wouldn't answer it. If a courier van brought something to the door, I wouldn't answer it. My anxiety would skyrocket and my heart would race.

The house felt cold and dark. The drives to and from Burnham were getting harder, and eventually I pushed for us to buy a house. I thought that would make everything better.

We found a bright blue 1950s house with yellow walls! It needed a lot of work, but I couldn't wait to get started on it. And it almost lifted my spirits a little bit. So we bought the house and took a week to strip it out while Mum and Dad looked after Jack. I was in heaven. It was the best feeling I'd had for so long. I was back in control!

Packing up and moving off the army base and into our own home for the first time felt so good. We worked hard to make it ours. And it had that new fresh paint and new carpet smell.

It didn't take long for reality to hit. Soon enough Dev was back at work, I was on my own again, and Jack was still crying. The hospital visits carried on. It didn't take me long to realise that, wherever we lived, all the old feelings were still there. And they weren't getting any better. Lots of people wanted to come over and see the new house and I struggled with that. It was becoming harder to put the happy face on. I even struggled to get to know the neighbour, Rosemary (who's an incredible person and is now my friend).

Moving in, I had a list of things that were going to get better and easier. It was better in many ways, but mentally I felt just the same. We'd done two moves within four months, so that had meant a lot of packing and unpacking and stress. But was I better? No.

If anything, I was more withdrawn. And the pressure was on Dev to help me get through the day. The air force was really supportive and let him work from home a lot of the time. I just needed to know he was there.

We'd moved Jack to another pre-school – and that meant fielding a lot of questions about whether or not I was working and what I liked to do in my free time. So I had to lie a bit. I didn't want to tell them that Jack was going to pre-school for my wellbeing, because then everyone would know. It was easier to lie. But of course, I wasn't going to work, so it still felt really difficult dropping him off in the morning.

All this time, Jack's health was getting worse, not better. He started to get ear infections every month or so, and his temperature spiked every time.

My appointment at the mothers and babies outpatients unit finally came through for November 2008. I was assessed by Dr Katy Brett, my psychiatrist registrar, and Gill Graham, a clinical nurse specialist. I saw a lot of Gill over the next few months and she was great.

I was horrendously nervous at the appointment. I had hot sweats and diarrhoea for three or four days beforehand. I was sure they were going to take my baby away and lock me up in a psychiatric hospital.

Devon came with me and we were met by a lady called Jean. She really made that little bit of time in the waiting room go by that much easier, and almost took my mind off things. There was so much information plastered over the wall in the waiting room – it was almost overwhelming. But Jean popped her head around the door and offered us a coffee and made sure we were okay.

A few girls went past: one was in a wheelchair and one had a feeding line. I thought they were mums. The image of that old mental hospital came up in my head again and I was genuinely scared. I didn't know any different at that stage, but the clinic was actually located next to the eating disorder unit.

We had a two-hour session with Dr Brett and Gill, and the last eleven months of struggling just came tumbling out my mouth. I was able to tell them lots, but I was still a little bit cautious, so I didn't tell them absolutely everything. I still had the lingering fear that they would lock me up and take Jack away.

There were a lot of tears, but that was okay. The more they listened, the more this weight began to lift from my shoulders. I still didn't know exactly what I needed back then but having someone to listen was a good start. And having someone to explain why this was happening and why I felt this way really helped. The sense of relief was enormous.

The next few visits with Gill were incredible. What an amazing lady! As time went by, I trusted her more and more. And that was so important for me. I wanted her to be Devon's mum – to be that paternal grandma figure to Jack. She was so empathetic and she really supported me. It made going there so much easier.

It was an eye-opener for me. I gained a new awareness of what makes me tick, and what makes me as a person. (I've learnt even more over the last nine years too.)

Jack continued to be checked by doctors and paediatrics staff. He had some more scans to check on the kidney stones which weren't showing any more, so we presumed they had finally passed.

It was coming up to Christmas and I felt that mix of stress and excitement. It was Jack's first Christmas and the excitement of the build up to the holidays overtook my own anxiety. Mum, Dad, Verity, and Marty were there, and it was so lovely to have my nana there too. I can see from the photos that I tried to look really happy on Christmas Day, but I wasn't. I was still pretending.

Jack was grizzly after our big Christmas dinner, so Dev put him to bed, and we carried on with our Christmas. Nana had made a very boozy trifle, and I was just putting the kiwifruit on the pavlova when I heard Devon calling from Jack's bedroom.

'Sonya, Sonya, come here!'

'Can't you wait a minute? I'm trying to cream this pav!' I shouted back at him.

'No, come here now,' he yelled down at me.

There was just something in his voice that made me stop ...

I ran to Jack's room and looked at him. He was purple, lifeless. He was lying on the floor, his head on one side, not breathing. It was the most horrifying thing I have ever experienced.

We started CPR and I called out to Marty to ring the ambulance. We finally managed to bring him round and he had a seizure. It was the longest time between Marty calling the ambulance and them arriving. It felt like a lifetime. I thought Jack was dying.

The ambulance crew got him stable. He seemed to be burning up, but his temperature was only 38.9 degrees. He was still purple and gasping for breath. And so, on Christmas night, we rushed my baby into hospital.

They explained that he was having a febrile convulsion. He would be okay for a bit, then have a convulsion and a spike in temperature and show the signs of becoming unwell again. And this wasn't a one-off – it became the new normal for us.

That was really hard to accept. It felt like a kick in the face. Like we were being told, 'Here: have something else to deal with!'

We sat in A&E for hours, and they finally managed to get his temperature down with a big hit of Pamol and ibuprofen. And then we discovered he had another infection. We were sent home six or seven hours later on Boxing Day morning.

Now we were on the alert for any change in Jack's temperature. We needed to check his temperature every hour – and that became our new norm for the next few weeks. With antibiotics, the ear infection cleared up in a couple of days, but we had to go on checking his temperature. It meant we had to send a thermometer and notebook with him to pre-school, and they would check it too.

We managed to get away for a weekend to Port Levy (a settlement on Banks Peninsula in Canterbury) with Mum, Dad, Verity, and Marty. We had a lovely couple of days. Jack didn't sleep – of course – but it was nice to get away.

But by the Monday, we noticed that something wasn't right with Jack. His temperature had started to creep up again, and there had been a little bit of blood in his urine. I couldn't get a doctor's appointment so we went to A&E, but the doctor just suggested we give him some paracetamol for kids and go home. So we arranged a follow-up doctor's appointment for the next day and left.

That night, Jack wasn't right at all. He was extremely restless and his temperature was creeping back up again. Now we could see some spots on him too – and they didn't fade under a glass. So we immediately started thinking: *meningococcal*.

Jack became sleepy as we waited in A&E, but eventually one of the senior paediatricians said we needed to head straight to the assessment unit. The young lady who was going to be looking after Jack was on duty by herself for the first time. I remember her coming over to us in her bright red stiletto shoes! She took some bloods and managed to get a few samples before his vein started to collapse and he went into full convulsion. It was the longest and worst convulsion we'd seen. It shocked everyone.

At one stage there were eight people in the room – from ICU staff to the high dependency unit staff to theatre staff – and they couldn't get a line in. His veins completely collapsed and he was in full seizure. Devon held him as they tried to get some anti-seizure medication in, but nothing was working.

I just couldn't handle it anymore. I had to leave the room with Devon. I was sick with worry. I couldn't believe what was happening, and I thought I was going to lose my little boy. He had only just turned a year old. It was so wrong.

And then, all of a sudden, it was as if something just clicked inside of me. I felt this bond, this rush of love wash over me. Everything suddenly flashed through my mind – the love, the fear and the uncertainty of what was happening in there ...

... And then suddenly one of the senior doctors came out and said it was time to make that phone call to our families. I didn't know what she meant. So she said, 'I'm sorry. Jack may not live.'

I felt sick to the stomach with grief. I went to the toilet and just vomited. When I came back, Devon was still standing there. He was white. I said we needed to ring Mum and Dad, but I couldn't even remember the number. It was as if my brain just switched off. I could feel myself starting to panic. It felt like I was having a heart attack.

Somehow, we managed to make the call. Everyone came straight over, and we just sat there in silence. People were going in and out of the treatment room and they were still trying to stabilise him. After around two hours they managed to get a line in through his foot and he finally stopped shaking. They needed to take a scan of his head to see what was happening in his little brain. They had the life packs on him, and we went down with him in the elevator.

It was the hardest thing I've ever had to do. I didn't think he was going to make it. I really thought he was going to die.

And as his mum, all this guilt that I hadn't loved my baby came flooding back. Only now, I knew how much I loved him. I finally felt that bond. I didn't want my little boy to die. I couldn't stop crying.

They asked us if we wanted to go in with Jack for his CT scan, and I just didn't know. But the nurse got us kitted out in big, heavy aprons and led us in. I remembered the machine from when Mum had had her cancer treatment when I was a little girl – and it was the same bloody machine! And now I was seeing my own child in it!

After the scan, they took us to the high dependency unit – intensive care for children – and they talked to us about doing a lumbar puncture. At this stage he was having a febrile convulsion but they still didn't know if it was part of the meningococcal reaction or not. I already knew how serious meningococcal was; I knew babies die from it.

Devon went with him for the lumbar puncture and the rest of us sat together, just waiting. Finally, the blood test came back – it wasn't meningococcal. The lumbar puncture results were fine too. And so they put the convulsions down to another virus. We spent seven days in hospital while they carried on monitoring him. The whole thing had been so scary. The only positive was that me and Devon were together.

Gill rang me from the mothers and babies unit a few times and even offered to come and see us – and I don't think that was part of her job description. But it was lovely to hear her voice on the phone. As usual, I said I was okay. I was trying to be really strong for everyone, but actually, I was at breaking point.

Dev and I took turns sleeping in the family room, while the other one would stay with Jack. It took a good three days for him to really come out of the sleepiness / seizure cycle. He was still hooked up on wires and monitors and being hydrated through a tube.

He had been so very unwell. The thought of losing him was massively distressing. I'll never forget that night – the thought of having to make that phone call still chills me. It makes me sick to think that the time I thought I was going to lose my child was the time I finally bonded with him.

Why had it taken twelve months – and why had it had to get that bad for me to feel bonded with Jack? I really struggled with that question and with all the guilt that went with it. I struggled with other things too – and they were only going to become apparent over the next few months ...

Kathryn: *"Why had it taken twelve months – and why had it had to get that bad for me to feel bonded with Jack?"*

Sonya's noticed something profound here. There are a multitude of potential "reasons" which could all be extremely valid answers to this question. Sometimes the incredible pain of not connecting with a baby we are desperate to connect with can lead us to spend hours on end coming up with reasons to explain it. Why now? Why not earlier? Why me? Why did this happen for my baby, for my family? Why did it have to be so hard?

Did that get your mind going? Did you find yourself caught up in those questions, whether it was for Sonya or for yourself or your loved one?

I invite you to consider this: do you think that noticing, recognising, knowing, and integrating the reasons why this has happened will really help you do what matters most to you?

Notice how this actually works, not what your mind tells you. Your mind will always tell you that more thinking is good! What does your experience actually tell you about what happens when all these questions show up? Can you ever be totally satisfied by the answers? And while you're busy thinking it through over and over again, aren't you missing out on something else?

In that sudden moment of presence and shock, Sonya connected with the profound truth: love and loss are flip sides of the same coin. If you don't desperately love someone, their loss can't hurt you. If loss threatens to hurt you incredibly, then you must know love. Sonya saw that coin stuck one way up: What if he dies? I can't lose him. I must keep him safe! *It's like being thrown into the deep end of the pool, rather than gently dipping a toe in like you would in a graduated exposure experiment. Sonya was given a sudden and intense exposure to the reality that Jack was going to die. That flipped the coin for her. She noticed what was right in front of her: love for her child.*

In a quite profound way, Jack had to almost die to be born for the first time in Sonya's heart. Our babies arrive to us at different points along the way. Some take longer than others. What if love isn't just what we feel in our hearts? What if it's something we do again, and again, and again, and again, and it moves us slowly in the direction of greater connection, compassion, and openness?

We all bring different experiences from our own history which can help or hinder motherhood. Sonya described how there were experiences in her childhood that highlighted some areas of vulnerability for her as she became a parent. That happens with many women.

In my work, it's really evident that becoming a parent is often the point at which past traumas can really emerge. Sonya's early experiences at the age of eleven – when she had to confront her mother's mortality – give us some clues as to why, later on, her own fears about dying and how to keep her baby alive were all the more urgent for her. Most mums are concerned with worries around keeping their baby alive and have an emerging sense of the massive responsibility that babies bring with them. In turn, this will then make them refer back to their childhood experiences with their own parents.

As Sonya says, she took on a lot of blame herself. She even thought she had caused things to go wrong for her mum in some way when faced with the possibility of her death.

As adults, we can look at this and know that she clearly had nothing to do with it. It was just chance. How could she possibly have caused it? And yet, when you think about it developmentally, that's precisely how a small child's mind works.

There's another point here that's really important to be aware of, particularly if you've had difficult and traumatic experiences in your own childhood. As children, the thing we need most from our parents or attachment figures is the knowledge that we can go to them for safety when we're in trouble. We need to know that we can depart from them and explore the world safely, coming back when we need help or to be soothed.

So what happens if our parents are unable to provide that reassurance for us and can't soothe us? They may be really scared themselves and convey their fears to us. Perhaps they're angry, and as a result we're scared to approach them. Or, as in Sonya's case, we might be afraid of them dying. In these cases, children are quick to look to themselves for what they might have done wrong. That's because children are entirely dependent on that adult figure for their own survival. This is part of what has helped humans evolve and stay alive over the course of hundreds of thousands of years. The difficulty is that the child in this scenario doesn't have the cognitive capacity to understand that things weren't their fault. But they've taken on that meaning very early on, partly because if they were to recognise how unavailable their parent was, the psychological distress associated with that would be very strong. So it's safer for them to see themselves as the problem.

If this has happened to you, just gently and kindly notice that it happened. Notice what you took away from that experience as a child and consider what you need now to help you feel safe and calm as you come into this phase of parenting.

Please also bear in mind that having these kinds of experiences doesn't automatically mean that you're going to suffer with postnatal depression, or that you're going to be in the same position as your own parents were. The cool thing is that humans are really good at adapting, and also there are other ways you can learn to soothe yourself and be safe in the world. But if you have a vulnerability, it is important to be aware of it. Then, as best as you can, you need to plan around that vulnerability and recognise what you need to do to reduce the risk of you becoming depressed.

If you experienced abandonment as a child, physically or psychologically, it's really normal for these terrors of abandonment to show up again as you move into the role of being a parent. That's not to say that they will definitely occur, and it's not to say would stop you from being the kind of parent you want to be. It may be that you just need to work a little bit harder, or plan for things a little bit differently. And that's what this book's here for.

CHAPTER 11

LETTING GO OF THE MASK

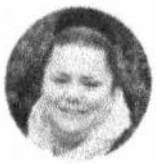

Sonya: The next couple of weeks after we took Jack home were pretty stressful. I was constantly watching his temperature. I got to a point where I was so tired of it that I just couldn't bring myself to do it anymore. I remember going to my outpatient appointment with Gill and blurting it all out to her. I think I was at my wits' end. I was mentally drained and so tired that I would have quite happily slept on the bathroom floor – anything to get a little bit of rest. I had a constant brain fog and I couldn't think straight. I felt like I'd done really well at holding it all together, but that day as I spoke to Gill, I just broke into a million pieces.

Gill talked to the registrar, who came in to see me. They told me I could stay in one of the rooms on the inpatient ward for a few nights, just to get some sleep. I burst into tears again; but this time through gratitude. It was just what I needed.

This was the reason they gave for my referral:

Mrs Watson was admitted to the ward with low mood, anxiety and a history of delayed bonding to her son, Jack. Jack has a significant medical history requiring several hospital admissions and a life-threatening febrile convulsion precipitated this admission. She had previously been managed as an outpatient for her depression but was struggling to cope at home and described extreme exhaustion and thoughts of driving herself into a bus. She was anxious and when Jack cried, this triggered fearful memories of the traumatic acts in A&E when Jack had his second febrile convulsion. Following the time Jack was in A&E being treated for the febrile convulsion and there were fears for his life, Sonya noted a change in her feelings towards him, becoming very positively attached thereafter.

Throughout Jack's life, sleep had been a challenging issue, exhausting everyone, and supporting a new way of managing this became one of the issues focused on during her admission.

I rang Dev to tell him I was going to be admitted. He went silent on the other end, but I told him it was going to be a good thing. I told him I was just going in for two or three days to get some sleep. All I could think about was the sleep! I remember thinking that I was going to feel like a million dollars after some rest. But I was still conscious that I was going to be admitted to a mental hospital – and that was scary. But actually, going there was one of the best things that happened in my life. And it wasn't scary at all; snuggled in against the Cashmere Hills, the hospital was an art deco style brick building with lovely gardens.

Besides, I was only going to be there for three days ...

Little did I know that those three days were going to turn into eight weeks, and that they were going to be the most important eight weeks of my life.

I had been diagnosed with a major depressive disorder (a single episode without psychotic features), acute stress disorder and delayed bonding to Jack.

I had twenty-four-hour nursing care and Jack slept down in the nursery, so I actually got some sleep! That was the best feeling ever. Devon came in to help me in the evening and the nurses took over after we tucked him up in bed. Jack still wasn't settling and was still crying, so the nurses put him on a sleeping programme. It was about six weeks until he was sleeping properly. Those nurses really were incredible. Without those people on the ward, I wouldn't be telling my story today.

I'd only really had one thought of suicidal intent, but I don't know how much worse it could have got. And so this really was an amazing eight weeks. It was during this time that I met Kathryn Whitehead, my inpatient psychologist. She was absolutely amazing, and I feel really privileged to be writing this book with her.

Kathryn taught me to let go of the mask. She taught me so much about who I was and where I was going. She helped me to manage what I needed to manage in my head. I really looked forward to my appointments with her. She really helped me through my journey.

Every Monday morning, I would have a meeting with everyone involved in my care to review my medication. I had to sit on the big orange seat – it was pretty intimidating! There were always six or seven people in the room, and I really felt anxious about how I should have been presenting the first few times. I was always offering my bed up to someone who needed it more, so at each meeting I didn't know if I would be sent home.

We had family meetings too. And they were hard, because, as Kathryn had told me, I had to take the mask off for those. It was only then that I found out that my mother had had postnatal depression, and so had my grandmother. My notes suggested that I "may have inherited a genetic predisposition to postnatal depression."

So maybe it was always going to happen, especially with all of Jack's health issues and the lack of support from Devon's parents ... there were lots of red flags on my postnatal journey. I think it's only around 2% of mothers that get to the inpatient care stage. I hadn't realised I was so unwell.

I didn't want to see any visitors, so I agreed with the staff that I wouldn't see anyone unless they'd rung through first. I didn't even want to go out in those first few weeks. I felt safe there. I really felt as if I could talk about what I was feeling, although it obviously took a little bit of time to break the wall down with Kathryn's help.

When I was on the ward, I worked on my brag book – it was a big clear file full of scrapbooking paper. We'd sit in a group in the mothers and babies unit and do a page on our thoughts and feelings every week.

From the first couple of weeks there are pictures of me sitting with Jack, and of course I'm smiling, because that's what I always did. But the words I wrote say how I was really thinking and feeling:

- Tiredness
- Anticipation
- Needing strength
- Why do I need to take medication?
- Lots of tears
- Masking it up
- How do I ask for help?
- Stress
- Sad
- Hate
- Feeling crazy
- Feeling drained

By week three and four, I was asking 'Why me?'

At least Jack was starting to sleep much better. We were getting him down within three or four minutes now, but I still felt tired. And even though we had established a connection, I felt as if I was still struggling to bond with him.

There are pictures in there of Jack waving to all the nurses and getting so many loving cuddles – something he missed out on a lot in his first year, if I'm being honest.

We went home for the first time in week five, and that felt a little bit strange after spending so long on the unit. My report showed that my mood had improved steadily and that, with advice and support, I was able to increase the time I spent with Jack. It read:

Sonya was seen for eleven sessions of Acceptance and Commitment therapy (ACT) by the ward clinical psychologist, Kathryn Whitehead. Two further sessions were offered to assist with the transition back to the outpatient team. Sonya entered treatment with a desire to learn how to relax and to come to terms with her grief about how different motherhood had been to her expectations. Sonya also wished to feel less burdened by constant anxious ruminations and memories of Jack's febrile convulsions (when she thought he would die). Sonya's high standards for herself, perfectionism, anger, and avoidance of her own emotions and experiences were major themes throughout therapy.

The early stages of therapy focused on identifying with Sonya ways in which avoidance of her internal experiences, and attempts to control these, had perpetuated her suffering. Mindfulness skills were practised at the start of each session to increase Sonya's ability to observe her own emotions and patterns of behaviour, with the added outcome of assisting her in her desire to "learn how to relax". The concept of acceptance was explored using a variety of metaphors, and Sonya worked on using willingness when faced with anxiety-provoking stimuli including Jack himself, family meetings and talking about her mental state. Cognitive diffusion skills were taught to assist Sonya to take her thoughts less literally and distance herself from them. She found it particularly helpful to use her creativity and artistic abilities when defusing from thoughts. Sonya created the metaphor of "Soup Mum", a figure who is opposite to Super Mum, by taking time out for herself, prioritising enjoying her children and leaving the house work undone. This was particularly helpful in regard to Sonya moving away from her perfectionist patterns. She explored her values, identifying being a good mum, communication, friendship, and love as important to her. Sonya then used her values to aid her in exposure tasks designed to address her anxiety and grief about Jack.

Final sessions focused on exposure work around Sonya's traumatic memories of the night she thought Jack would die of a febrile convulsion. Sonya was able to maintain her "observer stance" throughout this, reporting afterwards that the experience seemed more distant and less raw. Relapse prevention and self-therapy sessions were a focus towards the end of therapy. Sonya's self-reported depression symptoms moved from the severe range on the Beck Depression Inventory to the mild range through the course of her admission. Sonya was an impressive participant in ACT, devoting considerable time to her own recovery and demonstrating an amazing willingness to examine her own experiences.

CHAPTER 12

DEVON'S STORY

Sonya: By the time I was ready for discharge, I was feeling quite nervous about going back to "normal life." I was going over all the "what-ifs ..." in my mind – even though I'd worked really hard on that sort of catastrophic thinking in the unit.

Dev was really excited to have us back home. He had been such an amazing support, but I knew work would be calling him back to Wellington.

I had a meeting before I was discharged to talk about looking ahead with more confidence. The consultant psychiatrist, Debbie, asked me if I would be interested in the Postnatal Depression Family / Whanau* New Zealand Trust at some stage, and I absolutely felt like I would like to be part of something like that.

Walking out of the unit was very emotional for me. I almost felt a little bit empty. The team at the mothers and babies unit were my angels; they saved me and helped me through a really hard time. Even though I knew they were only a few minutes away, and I could call if I needed them, it felt as if my safety net just dropped away. I was going home and hoping for the best.

I knew that I'd shut my friends out. Luckily, they stayed by me and wrote letters to me. I think it took my family a long time to get their heads around where I was on my journey. It isn't easy to explain that journey and what it looks like to someone who hasn't had a mental illness. And it must have been hard for them; I had always been very good at putting that mask on. But once you take the mask off, it's pretty raw underneath. It isn't a nice thing to experience as a new mum.

*Whanau is the Maori word for family. It is a broad concept and can include close friends alongside extended family and friends of the family.

Within a month or so of me getting out of the inpatient unit, Devon went downhill. It was like looking at myself in the mirror, but this time it was Devon. I ignored it the first week, but it didn't get better. I could see the signs of sadness and the lack of empathy and emotion. He was still really helpful – he always was – but suddenly I felt like I'd lost him.

That was so hard. I was still trying to practise all the things I'd learnt from Kathryn. But I was so worried about Devon – and to what extent he was unwell. I even started to worry about the possibility of him taking his own life ...

We got him some help. He saw a psychologist who was incredible. And sure enough, it turned out he had postnatal depression. Lots of guys get it actually. I didn't even think about the possibility of Dev getting it when I was really unwell. At the time, I thought, *He's at work, he gets to come home and he's feeling good. He doesn't have to deal with the crying during the day* ... But it happened. It had all been stacking up inside.

I think a lot of his issues were around supporting me, but Jack had been unwell for so long and Dev was still dealing with his family wiping us out of their lives. It had been a huge roller coaster. We still feel the sadness that his parents haven't seen Jack since he was three weeks old. I often look at grandparents with their grandchildren and think how I would love them to be a part of my kids' lives. If I could put an ad up to find new grandparents, I would!

Like the doctors said in the unit, it's their loss that they don't get to spend time with our kids. But obviously this was a huge thing for Dev to deal with.

He started on medication, saw a psychologist, and had a great response.

This is his side of the story ...

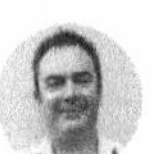

Devon: Like any first-time dad, I felt elated and excited when Sonya told me the news ... and a little bit nervous too. We had been trying for a while and of course we had all the normal anxieties: was everything going right with the pregnancy?

I tried to make it to most of the midwife appointments, and the pregnancy went really well. There was that stage when the scan showed cysts on the brain that obviously worried us. So we used "Doctor Google" to find out what it was, and we tried to be prepared for the worst-case scenario. That certainly added to the pressure, but then, when the next scan showed that they'd gone, we felt a huge surge of relief.

I wasn't aware of any concerns that Sonya had as a first-time mum, apart from the obvious nerves. And things went well right up to the end of the pregnancy.

My eye injury occurred around Sonya's thirty-eight or thirty-ninth week of pregnancy. Add that to Sonya's dad's stroke and an overdue baby, and the pressure was really on us. I knew Sonya was struggling. I was pretty much useless. I was bedridden for the first week or so, and then I remember Sonya pushing me around in a wheelchair to see an optometrist while she was forty+ weeks' pregnant.

I felt a lot of guilt – I couldn't believe I'd done this at the time when Sonya really needed me the most. It was so hard. We did get some assistance from Sonya's sisters which was a huge relief, and Caroline was there with us during the birth. They were fantastic.

I was still meant to be resting; I was there at the hospital, but I couldn't really do much. I wasn't even meant to drive but I ended up driving anyway, just so I could be around for Sonya.

Being at the birth was awesome. It was great just to see Jack come out and see that he was healthy. And it was such a relief to see Sonya get through it okay. I remember us going into recovery late at night and then making our way back to the ward. Sonya was in the bed and couldn't really move much because of her C-section. We had talked a bit about it, and we were somewhat prepared for what would happen, but the surgery came with its own issues.

That first night everything seemed okay, until we were back in the room and Sonya couldn't move. The ward was full, and there were only two nurses on. Sonya had to ring a bell if she needed help, but no one would come. I was disgusted to be told to leave that first night. It meant Sonya pretty much had to cope by herself, but of course she couldn't, because she couldn't move. That obviously put a whole lot of pressure on her.

My own experience of parenthood in those first few days was different. I particularly remember sharing the experience with Joe – another dad from the antenatal class. They'd had twins earlier on the same day we'd had Jack. So we were all in the hospital together. At one stage, the two of us were in the corridor just crying away, just so happy to be dads. It was an awesome feeling to have Jack in our lives.

I was totally unaware of the thoughts that were going through Sonya's head as she was trying to recover from her C-section, trying to breastfeed, and trying to get that bond with Jack.

I probably felt that I had an immediate bond with Jack; but I had lots of opportunities to hold him and he would fall asleep on my chest. It was so much harder for Sonya. She had the tubes, the drain, the breast pumps, the pain from her C-section, and the problem with the circulation in her legs. She was in no fit state to have that time with Jack. So while I took that first week in my stride, Sonya would have related to the experience differently, with all the pressure that was on her. Looking back, all I had to do was be there.

Seeing Sonya in so much pain was hard – why was it happening to her? One of the other ladies on the ward had had a C-section with a different doctor. She was up and walking around within a couple of days, whereas Sonya was still struggling with all the pain. It extended her recovery period and made everything that much harder.

The reflux diagnosis didn't help either. It didn't have as much of an impact the first few days when we were trying to get breastfeeding established ... who knew it was going to become such a big problem! The first night home, we were sitting on the couch in Jack's room and he just wouldn't stop crying. We tried bottle-feeding him and he just vomited it up. We were so worried he wasn't getting enough to eat, so we fed him some more and he vomited that up too. It was just a vicious cycle. And the two of us sat there with him crying, asking ourselves, 'What have we done? Why have we been lumped with a baby like this?' We talked about it endlessly, wondering if there'd been a reason why a baby like Jack had been given to us.

I remember walking around our housing area trying to get him to stop crying. I would think, *Why us? Why is Jack like this? Why isn't he a normal baby?* But in the end, we knew we just needed to be loving parents and help him through this.

In the first week, he was too big for his crib, so he ended up in his cot in his own room. He didn't get a chance to be close to us in the bedroom for any length of time, which most babies do get.

When I got back to work, I got lots of advice from the ladies at work, but it was all conflicting. Some of it was totally against what Plunket would tell you. So I never quite knew what the right thing to do was.

One night, two or three weeks after getting Jack home – two or three weeks of no sleep for any of us – we ended up taking him back in to see the paediatrician. His reflux was just so bad, he wasn't taking anything down. And I remember the paediatrician holding him for over an hour, just trying to get him to calm down. He told us how his kids had had reflux too – and they'd had it until they were three years old! Up to that point, everyone had been telling us that we'd be all right in a few months.

That night the paediatrician sent us home to rest while they looked after Jack in the hospital. I know it was the doctor had the best intentions, but we felt so guilty. As I drove home, I thought to myself that I needed to turn around and go and get him. As parents, it just didn't seem right to leave him there. In the end, it did help to get a night's rest and recharge the batteries a little bit.

We had made a conscious decision to have a family, and Jack was just Jack. He was ours. We needed to find a way to get through what he was going through. We learnt a lot over that time about reflux and different medications. Sonya had a meticulous approach to writing down the doses and the timings to make sure we got everything right for him.

The guilt was hard on us. I knew Sonya felt it. We were both wondering if this was what it was really like to be a parent. And I guess I just kept on thinking, *One more week* ... Everyone would tell us to just get to one month, and then two months, and then three months ... I was looking at those dates and hurdles and thinking, *If we can just get through to this date or that date, it will be better ...*

But soon we realised that things weren't getting better; they were only getting worse. Asking for a transfer to Christchurch was a big call – but I believe it was the right one. Blenheim was a lovely place to live, and we had great friends and a really awesome antenatal group, but no family at all. As Sonya mentioned, we had a big falling out with my parents and my mum wrote us off. Sonya's parents were in Christchurch and their travel was limited, so we didn't have that close family support that a lot of families get. We thought moving to Christchurch was the right decision. I got mixed responses from my military commanders. Surprisingly, my male commanders were more supportive than my immediate commander, who was a female. The males were telling me I had to do what was right for my family, whereas the female response was, 'Well, I've had babies and I got through it, and so will Sonya.'

It was hard to say goodbye to the house at Woodburn just four months after Jack had been born. It was our first family home. But it felt like the right thing to do.

Unfortunately, it didn't turn out that way and it ended up making things a lot worse. The army camp had a different feel to it, the house was filthy, and Sonya felt isolated. It didn't help that I now had to commute and travel quite a bit. So while I was busy at work, Sonya was stuck in this dirty, filthy house surrounded by people she didn't know. She felt just as far away from her parents as if she was still in Blenheim. We felt like we'd made a big mistake.

I was always concerned about going back to work. I'd had a few weeks at home but felt like I hadn't been able to support Sonya properly. Jack's health issues meant that Sonya couldn't take Jack to all the groups and sessions that everyone else was able to go to. She just couldn't take Jack into those situations.

Travelling into Christchurch to see paediatricians and doctors and for various appointments was like a full-time job. That was another aspect of living out there that made things hard for Sonya. I could see her going downhill and I felt guilty because I'd been travelling away so much.

When we were in Blenheim I'd obviously had a few concerns about Sonya's mood and I'd spoken to a midwife. But in Christchurch I didn't know who to call. The midwife had run through the Edinburgh scale with her (a screening measure for postnatal depression), but Sonya – being Sonya – could see the scores and knew what answers she needed to give to come out on the good side of the scale.

Later, Sonya got on to the Postnatal Adjustment Programme and had home visits. She'd seen the GP, she was on medication ... and I thought that all meant she was on the road to recovery. But nothing seemed to work, and it still got worse. And we still had all of Jack's health issues and the sleep deprivation to deal with.

Sonya didn't really talk to me much about how she was feeling. I would ask her and she'd tell me she was okay, and then tell me to go to work. So I would. But in retrospect, it was clear she had her mask on.

I probably did the normal guy thing and assumed everything was good. Or I'd tell her all the practical things she could do to make herself feel better: go out for a walk and get some fresh air. Do this and do that ... the normal "blokey" thing of trying to fix it with practical suggestions. I was going about it totally the wrong way obviously; I wasn't allowing her to find what she needed to do.

There were times when she told me that she just wanted to give up; she didn't feel like doing this anymore. I would just try to provide some positive encouragement. Perhaps I didn't take it seriously enough. There were times when she'd been driving and she said she had just wanted to drive into the back of a truck or into a tree, and again maybe I didn't take it seriously enough. I just tried to offer encouragement and what I thought were good solutions. There was probably a degree of anger and frustration on my part: the frustration that nothing was getting better. We'd moved across the country. Why weren't things changing? What were we doing wrong? What hadn't I found out that I needed to do to help? It was not a very good time.

One of the times I really knew something was up was when I left Sonya on the couch in her PJs in the morning, then came home later to see that she was still there. She hadn't done anything. She hadn't showered, and it wasn't like Sonya to just sit there doing nothing. But her motivation was gone.

You don't know as a first-time dad. You don't know what the signs are unless you've gone through it, or you've been with someone who's gone through postnatal depression before. You don't know what you need to do when you get to that point. You just try to carry on working your way through it. Looking back at it now, the solution just seems so obvious. But that's with hindsight, and that's knowing the triggers.

It was scary when Sonya was admitted to the mothers and babies unit, but it was also a huge relief. I knew Sonya was getting the help she needed. And then, when Sonya came home, it was like having the old Sonya back! She was still on the road to recovery, but you could really see that the old Sonya was on her way back after fourteen or fifteen months.

At this point, I thought, *Okay, we've got there, now I can relax*. But that's when things started to hit me, and I started to go downhill. Everything that I'd been going through finally caught up with me. The key point I'll always remember is getting Jack into the car seat and I just couldn't buckle the seat up. I went absolutely off my tree. I was swearing and poor little Jack was in the seat looking at me, alarmed, wondering what he'd done wrong.

I just had to walk away, and straightaway Sonya asked me if I needed help. And I knew I did.

So I went and saw the military doctor on the camp and he was really good. Then I went to see a counsellor and we talked through the whole thing that had happened with Sonya. But I also got to talk about the situation with my mum, and about all my feelings after falling out with her.

It was a positive process. It helped me get to the point where I focused entirely on my family. Mum and Dad were the ones missing out; I had to concentrate on Sonya and Jack. I put the focus entirely on us – and that was probably the best decision I made.

The counselling really helped, and I stayed on medication for about eighteen months. I went to a PNAP event (that's a group treatment for PND: the Postnatal Adjustment Programme) with other partners of women going through postnatal depression. It was really good to talk about our own experiences. It helped us be more aware of PND itself, and of how to help our partners. That really gave me the energy to give a little bit back. We joined the Postnatal Depression Family / Whanau New Zealand

Trust, initially in an advisory role. But over the last five or six years, we've been board members. Sonya facilitates support groups, and I've been secretary, treasurer, and now Chair. We're basically giving back to all the other people in the community who need help.

A few years after Jack was born, we made the decision to try for another baby. For a time, we'd thought we wouldn't have any more children, but it was entirely different this time. When Lily arrived, everyone was so much more aware of all the issues; Sonya's history was all flagged up on her file and we had an excellent midwife. It was amazing how different the treatment was. We got through that *and* we got through the earthquakes!

You don't wish this kind of experience on anyone, but ... we wouldn't know anything about PND if we hadn't gone through this journey for ourselves. We wouldn't be in a position to help others and we wouldn't be here to talk to dads and families. We wouldn't be involved in running support groups for mums who are going through this experience.

Even though I wouldn't want to do it again, the experience and what I have learnt from it has been positively life-changing.

CHAPTER 13

THE HEALING ROAD

Sonya: I'd come a long way and made a lot of progress but recovering from postnatal depression takes time. It doesn't happen overnight. Looking back, it probably took a couple of years before I really felt like I was recovered.

The first part of my recovery was definitely having some community support in place. For me it was Stepping Stones: I had a community support worker for six to seven months. She'd come and see me every week and we'd talk about all sorts of things. She provided such great support.

I also had help from Parents as First Teachers (PAFT) and they came monthly to help me with Jack's milestones. The paediatric team continued to support me with his ongoing health issues. I kept going to the mothers and babies outpatients unit for another couple of months until May, when I was discharged. My neighbour Rosemary was absolutely brilliant too.

I was using my own self-help tools more and more – one of the most important ones for me was learning to accept the fact that I needed to take medication, and that was okay.

We were also asked to be an advisor for the Family / Whanau New Zealand Trust. After we'd had our first advisor's meeting, I was asked to fly up to a conference in Wellington and give a presentation about myself and my journey. That was only about five months on from coming out of inpatients, so it was pretty incredible. Being able to volunteer my time back to the trust was a huge part of my healing.

I think my outlook on life changed a lot in terms of what I wanted from life and what I was going to do next. And that's all thanks to Jack. If I hadn't had Jack I wouldn't be doing what I'm doing now. Eight years on, I'm still working as the coordinator / facilitator for PND Canterbury www.pndcanterbury.co.nz. I pushed to start a support group five or six years ago. At the very first meeting, without any advertising, we had eight mums turn up just from word of mouth. We didn't have any childcare; it was just me and the mums and it was absolutely crazy! But five years on it's a fully facilitated support group. I coordinate it all, and we have Cassie, our volunteer / childcare facilitator to help us. We also have a team of volunteers that come and help out each week. It's wonderful to have the opportunity to help all these mums and build up such a close rapport. We have helped hundreds and hundreds of mums.

It really has been an incredible journey – and I feel really privileged to be a part of other parents' journeys. We talk about everything in our groups, things like self-care, self-help, stigma, meal planning, the pressures of sex after having a baby (with postnatal depression, anxiety or bipolar), and so much more.

I wrote the programme and it covers everything I learnt on the mothers and babies unit. It involves lots of self-help, together with specialist treatment – at the end of the day, that's what works. But first of all, it's so important that people accept the fact that postnatal depression is very real. And everyone's journey is different. I think that people tend to forget that. What happened to me probably wouldn't happen in the same way with someone else. It's about accepting your journey for what it is. It would be amazing if we had a magic wand, but we can't change that journey. However, doing the work I do now – and doing this book – has made it an amazing one.

I know that if I can share my story – even if it's with just one other person – then my job is done. And that has been a huge part of my healing process for PND and anxiety.

I really didn't think we would try for a second child, but yes, we did.

I was adamant throughout my journey that I wouldn't want to have another baby. But prior to my postnatal depression, we'd always talked about having two or three children. And in the end, time heals.

We found out we were pregnant in 2010, with a due date (again) of January. We put lots of good things in place – I was a lot more aware of my mood and my mental state. Jack was nearly three and still having paediatric support, but our day-to-day life with him was now very different ...

Jack was two years old when I was pregnant with our second child. At this stage, he was still pretty much non-verbal – he could really only say "Mum" and "Dad" – and he stayed non-verbal until he was three years old. We had lots of different support services in place for him; we had the Ministry of Education, who helped us with his speech, behaviour, and sensory issues. We had support from an occupational therapist from Beacon House out at Burwood who helped Jack with his coordination. Even though he wasn't actually diagnosed with Sotos syndrome until he was seven, there were very clear signs of it – he was very clumsy, his fine motor skills hadn't developed, and he experienced lots of sensory issues. He still couldn't walk or talk, and he experienced very high anxiety. He did have a little bit of anger there too, and we were slightly concerned that he might hurt the new baby, so we put a plan in place for that too.

A lady called Sue came in Monday to Friday, from four to five o'clock, to help with his bath and his evening feed. He was still quite a difficult toddler. Sometimes he would thump his head against the wall, which we found hard to deal with. We were still juggling lots of hospital appointments, so life with Jack continued to be pretty exhausting. But we loved him so much. And the benefits of all that extra support really paid off further down the line. Now, Jack is nine years old – and he is such a beautiful child.

When I was pregnant, we tried to explain to Jack that we had a baby coming. We encouraged him to help us set up the baby's room. We got lots of books out of the library to try to explain the concept to him.

The pregnancy was great. At the twenty-week scan, we found out we were having a girl, and everything looked really good. Everything went smoothly, apart from the earthquake in Christchurch that damaged our house.

It's hard for anybody – let alone a little boy with global development issues – when your house starts to crack and windows pop. That obviously triggered his anxiety, and when he saw the liquefaction he thought it was like worms coming out of the earth. But we made sure to tell him that whatever happened, no matter how many worms came up, we would always be there to keep him safe.

After that, things were fine all the way up to Christmas Eve 2010 ...

I couldn't feel a lot of movement from the baby, and I ummed and ahed about what to do. It was such a busy time of year ... but I couldn't feel much movement, so I rang my midwife. Liz was incredible and she told me to come on up to the hospital so they could check me out.

My midwife put me on the monitor. She looked and listened and then said, 'I'll just be a minute ...' She popped out and came back with a senior doctor.

'Hmm, not a lot of movement going on,' he said. 'Let's get you in for a C-section.'

The baby was thirty-six weeks old at this stage, and I was going in for an emergency C-section on Christmas Eve. I couldn't believe it.

In no time at all we were in the theatre and I had an epidural put in. Devon and the midwife were there and the theatre staff were brilliant. They started cutting, but they really struggled to get through all the scar tissue from the first C-section. So much so that they had to call in the senior doctor.

It was such a mess. Adhesions had connected to my kidneys and my bowel. The doctor said it looked as if a chainsaw had gone through there. So all the pain I'd had after my C-section with Jack – all the buzzing bees – hadn't been in my head. It had all been real. So real that the doctor told me he would never want to see me in there having a C-section ever again.

After a good fifty minutes of cutting they found that my baby had got stuck, so they had to use forceps to remove her. That's something they don't normally do, so it marked her face quite a bit. She came out not breathing. She was purple.

I was lying there waiting. The anaesthetist kept saying, 'Wait, your baby will cry ...' and I all I could do was keep waiting and waiting. My anxiety was through the roof. But my baby didn't cry. They continued to work on her, the anaesthetist trying to reassure me. She was telling me my baby was going to be all right, but there was no sound ...

Finally, a little cry came out. I let out a huge sigh of relief.

They gave her oxygen and started working on her chest. Devon cut the cord and she finally came round. She was placed straight onto my chest for a very short time. It was the most amazing feeling ever. I can't even explain it ... just incredible. I only wish that I'd had that experience with Jack, as things might have been different. We called our little girl Lily.

Lily's temperature and blood sugar levels were still really low, so they took her away and put her in an incubator. *Oh my goodness, here we go again*, I thought.

The neonatal unit (NICU) was full, so she stayed with me and we were transferred into recovery. The paediatric team checked on her every twenty minutes. I was talking to a lovely Scottish nurse in the recovery area. She was taking some colostrum off my breast and was pulling it up in the syringe to give to Lily. As she was getting the air out of it, she squirted it up to the ceiling. It was such a funny moment, and it was so good to just be able to laugh. It was such a contrast to my experience with Jack.

It meant so much that I was able to touch Lily through the incubator. That made such a difference. I could see her at all times, and I had as much help with her as I needed.

We stayed in Christchurch Women's Hospital. Thanks to my midwife and the mothers and babies unit, I was given an extended stay of seven days, plus extra time if I needed it. What a complete difference! I was so well supported. I was still on my medication which made me quite sleepy, so the nurses on the ward would take Lily at night so that I could get some sleep.

They helped me with the breastfeeding, and I got plenty of rest, so it felt like a real turning point in my journey. I had had two completely different birth experiences, my second one obviously being a lot more positive. And I thank the staff for that.

My C-section healed within one week! There were no ongoing health issues. My mental status was so much better, even though we had a Boxing Day earthquake in the hospital. My midwife was so well educated on postnatal depression and anxiety, and was constantly asking me how I was feeling. I had my first post-birth appointment at mothers and babies, so everything was put in place for me.

It felt lovely going home this time too, and I was even able to go on working from home for the Trust. It was an incredible experience. The bond I had with Lily was immediate, even though I'd had an emergency C-section. And even though she was born at thirty-six weeks, she still weighed in at 8lb 14oz! All of these things made my second journey so much better than my first.

There was another earthquake in February and our house basically broke, so we had to stay with friends for eight weeks. But actually, it was a really wonderful time. No one could work, so we were all at home. It felt like that old idea of a community raising a baby. That's what used to happen, and it doesn't happen now – unless there's an earthquake! There were four adults in the house, two young children and Lily. It was a totally different experience – and possibly the thing that helped keep me clear of postnatal depression.

It was probably a bit harder for Jack though! He could be pretty trying at times. After we got home we had to keep Lily's bassinet in the lounge area so I could see where they both were. He was a bit sneaky though and would try to push the bassinet over with her in it. Sometimes he would just take off down the road, so we were always on high alert for Jack's safety and wellbeing.

Jack's vocabulary really started to develop after Lily was born. By the time he turned three, he already looked like a five or six-year-old because he was so big and tall. He was very often mistaken for an older child. So if he was having a meltdown in the supermarket, people's expectations were that he should be behaving himself because he was five or six, but actually he was still only three years old! I did feel judged, but I've got to the point now where I don't really care what other people think. People think they have a right to judge parents and open their mouths and say exactly what they think – but that can be absolutely devastating for most mums and dads. Deep down inside, most of us take that to heart.

I've learnt, with Jack being so big, to be more relaxed about it all. I think, *Hey, he's got Sotos syndrome, and he's still such a beautiful child*, so we're at the point where we just ignore any comments about his height and his size. And now, of course, Jack knows all about his Sotos syndrome. It's actually benefitted him with his sports, especially his basketball and swimming. Things could be a lot worse.

CHAPTER 14

YOU ARE NOT ALONE

Sonya: It's not easy to finish my story. I've started writing this so many times. I talk about these things with mums every day, but I think I've struggled with bringing my own story to a close because in some ways, it really does feel like the end of the journey. And it's been more emotional than I was expecting; I've gone into more detail than I would at conferences. It's exposed a lot of raw emotion and brought some of that old anxiety back.

Unfortunately, postnatal depression will never go away in the world. There's never going to be a permanent fix. But I think that we, as a community and as parents, need to break the stigma. We need to break the silence around mental health, antenatal depression and postnatal depression. We need to help support our mums and our dads and our families because it's a road that no mother or child should ever have to travel alone, without support, love, empathy, and understanding. They should always be supported.

I think that we're starting to get there, but we've still got a long way to go. We need to be able to ask a mum those important questions: 'Hey, how are you doing? Are **you** okay? I'm not asking about the baby now – are you okay?' We need to be prepared for the answer. As you'll have read, it was really tempting to put that mask on and say, 'Yeah, I'm coping.' But actually, deep down inside, I wasn't coping at all.

Thank God Kathryn could see through that. And from time to time I know that I still put that mask on, but I try to avoid that as much as possible.

This process has shown me that we need to spread understanding about mental health. It's okay to have mental health issues in a family. So we – as a community, as a country, and as a world – need to support our families when they're going through this. And really, it's quite easy to do. The mums that I see each week reach out for support, but it would be so much better if they'd known they could have reached out sooner. Wouldn't it be so much better if new mums and dads started out on this journey knowing that it is okay to ask for help?

You don't need to be brave. You don't need to put on your mask. You don't even need to be a Super Mum. There are services out there that can help. I know that a lot of these services would benefit from more funding – like anything to do with mental health. But there are people out there who will listen. And they *will* help.

If you're reading this because you're worried about a new mum, then take the time to ask her if she's okay. Look her in the eye and be prepared for the answer that she's not coping. We can't know what goes on behind closed doors at home. It can be such a lonely experience, sitting at home by yourself, day in and day out.

And if you're a new mum, please – never compare yourself to anyone else. Never compare your journey with anyone else's. Everyone will have a different experience. Your baby could be amazing – it could sleep and feed really well – and yet you still might not feel well. You might still feel like crying a lot of the time. Maybe you can't cope with the change in routine and the change in lifestyle. It is a huge transition when you a baby, whether it's your first baby or your fourth baby. It's still a huge change. And change is hard to deal with for everyone involved ...

So please, please do ask for help. This is something you don't have to do alone.

PART II

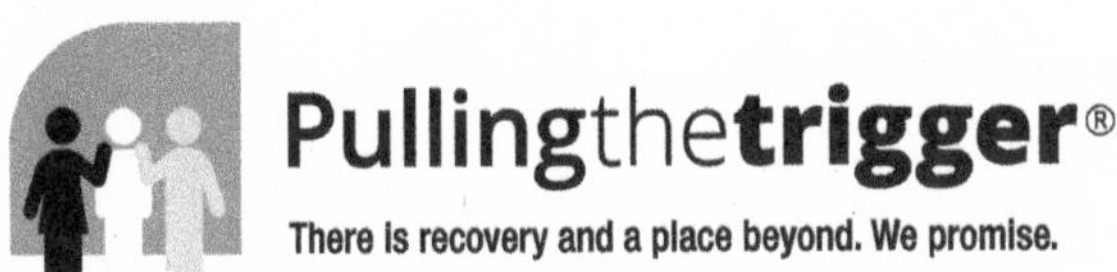
Pullingthetrigger®
There is recovery and a place beyond. We promise.

The Definitive Treatment and Recovery Approach

I couldn't be a good mother, I didn't know how. Kathryn was my saviour, someone that could put me on the right path. Embrace this approach, like I did, and embrace a new future with your baby. Your journey is about to begin.

Sonya Watson

SECTION 1

BALANCING THE IMPOSSIBLE

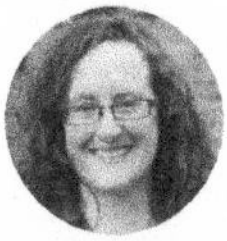

Kathryn: Motherhood can be like walking a tightrope over Niagara Falls. Think of that massive waterfall and the crashing sound of the water. Imagine the feel of the spray on your face and the slight giddiness in your stomach as you peer cautiously over the edge. Some days there is so much mist at Niagara that it's hard to see very far in front of your face. The sound of roaring water is screaming in your ears. And you have to walk a tightrope over this?!

Too late. Once you're pregnant you're already one or two steps across before you even know it.

This journey can be terrifying. But that's motherhood! On one side is your baby, on the other side are your own needs. You've got baggage with you too. As you set out into the mist, inching out across the rope with a large balancing pole in your hands, everything is unpredictable. It feels as if you have no control, and you're working hard to balance your baby and your own needs.

Motherhood often feels like something you've got to do entirely on your own. Just like Niagara, sometimes the environment makes it feel harder than at other times. Niagara can feel so different when it's particularly windy, or if it's been raining and the falls are full. This is rather like how some environments are harder to mother in than others.

Of course, for some people it's not like Niagara Falls at all; the course of motherhood might just be like a small, peaceful stream. While it's certainly awesome when that happens, I'm guessing that's not your experience, and that's not why you're reading this book.

Environmental conditions can change, but the hard part is that you've got very little control over whether they change or not. We

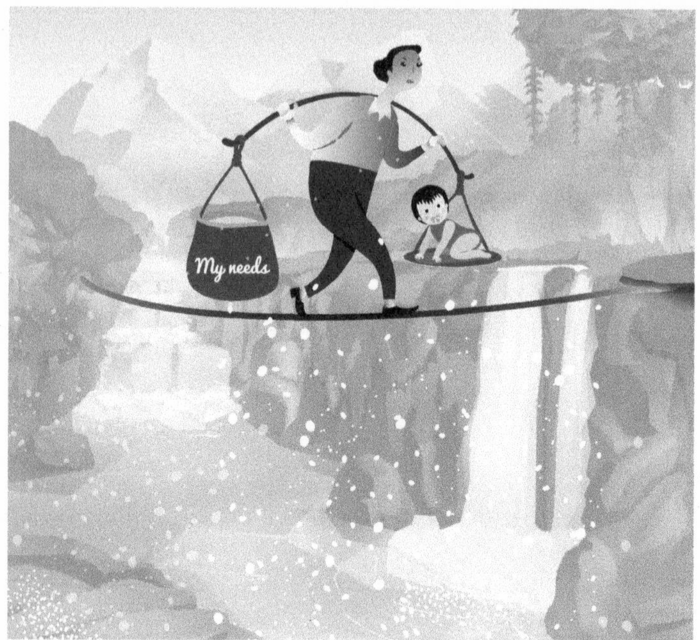

***Figure 1:** Balancing the needs of you and your baby.*

bring all our history with us to this task of motherhood. It's our backpack. Sometimes our backpack might feel neatly and evenly packed so that it's easy for us to balance. Other times, it will feel uneven and wonky – full of all the bits of our history that we don't want to look at anymore. Other times, our pack is messy and untidy, so that the contents fall out along the way.

Our focus also makes a difference. If we're lucky, we'll find a balance where we can concentrate on each step, aware of the rope, the wind, and the destination. Other times, there'll be a cloud of thoughts around our head – like the swirling mist, distracting us. It feels as if our mind is pulling us one way or the other. Our destination is entirely unclear. Where on earth are we going? Sometimes we can't work out who we are, or what our needs are. Sometimes babies bring with them their own challenges, and particular needs that are hard to meet as we struggle across the tightrope.

I see motherhood as a journey of great courage. In many ways, it's an everyday miracle and often underappreciated by the rest of the population.

In an ideal world, if you were going to learn how to walk a tightrope, you'd probably begin with a rope across the ground and practise walking along that. Then you'd attach a rope between two trees and practise that way. But what about motherhood? If you're lucky, you'll have already had the opportunity to practise with babies, to learn what babies are like, and to understand that if a baby wants or needs something, it can't be delayed, even if you don't know what that need is straightaway.

If you're unlucky, though, it'll feel like getting onto the tightrope with no practise at all. This isn't your fault, it's just how our current society is set up. One of the things that probably makes tightrope walking a little bit simpler (if it can ever be considered simple) is having a safety net – and you can stitch one for yourself ...

Your mothering safety net is your social support – the people that can be there to set you right when you wobble, or even catch you when you fall. Building up those social supports and then reaching out to them often requires overcoming a whole set of barriers, including your own sense of shame, the feeling that maybe you've failed at this amazingly important job, and the belief that you should be able to do it all on your own.

And then there are all the comparisons we make: we compare what we feel on the inside with what everyone else shows on the outside. Women can look confident while holding down a job, parenting several children, keeping their relationship going, and having a perfect house! We often compare that to our own feelings of hopelessness and helplessness, and we find ourselves wanting.

If you have any feelings of anxiety, depression or trauma emerging, that will make it even more difficult for you to reach out to others. But reaching out will help you to build that safety net. One of the many opportunities that babies bring us is the chance to be vulnerable and to take new risks.

And I'm hopeful that this book will help you to do that.

SECTION 2

BEFORE YOU START ... STOP!

Now, I know you're probably raring to go, but, just before you begin working through this book, I'd encourage you to pause and ask yourself: *Is there space for me to do this right now?* At any time you can choose to stop or continue doing what you've always done. You don't have to do anything this book suggests. Everything is an invitation.

SAFETY

If you are struggling with thoughts of suicide, you feel as if you're preoccupied by death, or you're on the edge of hurting your baby or child, I urge you to get immediate help. Go and call your local mental health crisis service, see your doctor, or ask someone you trust to help you. Stop reading and do it right now. The safety of yourself, your children and others always comes first.

Remember what they say in the aeroplane? Whose oxygen mask should you fit first? That's right: yours. Your baby relies on you to keep them safe. Emotional wellbeing is the same. If you can't take care of yourself enough to put your own emotional oxygen mask on, you're unlikely to be able to take care of what your baby needs. So if it's not something you've learnt before, I invite you to begin learning how to administer self-care now.

TRAUMA

I'd particularly encourage you to stop before you start if you've got a history of trauma. By that I mean very scary things happening where your life or your safety was under threat, or the life or safety of somebody else. Some examples of this might be birth trauma, where you were worried that you or your baby would die, or early childhood trauma like sexual abuse. There's a much higher chance that issues relating to this trauma will emerge in postpartum. I'd encourage you to use your suffering as a way of understanding whether or not it's worth going ahead and proceeding with the exercises in this book.

Ask yourself: *Is the cost of suffering, or not working on these issues, higher than the cost of taking the time to address it?*

Always remember that, at any time, you can choose to stop, or just keep going back to doing what you've always done. You might also want to find an ally, someone you trust to help you work through the exercises. Another important thing to keep in mind is that even if there is trauma in your history, you don't necessarily have to go back and dredge it all up if you're not ready. Healing doesn't inevitably involve pushing at your barriers and having to recall what's happened.

PACE YOURSELF

I'd really encourage you to work through this book at a pace that works for you. I encourage this because I know how hard it is when you push yourself, and I know that sometimes, people push themselves too hard without even realising they're doing it. If you realise that you're pushing too hard, then I'd suggest perhaps doing half of what you think you can do, then pausing and stopping and seeing how it's working for you. It can be really helpful to know that different kinds of help are needed depending on how stressed or low you feel. We know that human brains get overwhelmed at a certain level of stress, and our capacity to think through what to do can go off-line at these times. Here's a help sheet on levels of arousal and coping strategies to guide you.

LEVELS OF AROUSAL AND SELF-SOOTHING

Keep in mind that brilliant proverb: a journey of a thousand miles starts with just one step. One step is all you need to take. It can be a very small step, or it can be a very large step. In this process, your awareness and self-observation are your friends.

Stop and notice now what it's been like reading these words ...

How do you feel in your body? What emotions are showing up for you? What have you got an urge to do? Perhaps you want to put this book down, perhaps you even want to throw it

<table>
<tr><th>Zone</th><th>How strong is the feeling?
1= not at all, 10 = very</th><th>Coping and Self-Soothing</th></tr>
<tr><td rowspan="3">Uncomfortable and Unmanageable
PAUSE (BE AWARE)</td><td>10</td><td rowspan="3">Push, then pause! In most cases, you'll want to bring your level of arousal down – it's not possible to think clearly at this level.
Use self-soothing and grounding.
Ask others for help. Focus on BEING SAFE.
My Ideas:</td></tr>
<tr><td>9</td></tr>
<tr><td>8</td></tr>
<tr><td rowspan="4">Uncomfortable and Manageable
OPEN</td><td>7</td><td rowspan="4">This is the zone to work in – pushing yourself slightly beyond comfort, so that you can grow and learn. Use mindfulness, acceptance, and valued action as you do this. Focus on DOING and BEING PRESENT.
My Ideas:</td></tr>
<tr><td>6</td></tr>
<tr><td>5</td></tr>
<tr><td>4</td></tr>
<tr><td rowspan="3">Comfortable and Manageable
ENGAGED</td><td>3</td><td rowspan="3">Mmm. A nice zone to be in. It's much easier to learn using words and ideas in this zone. If you're working on challenging yourself, make sure you spend plenty of time doing things to chill out and feel relaxed.
Stay engaged in life. ENJOY!</td></tr>
<tr><td>2</td></tr>
<tr><td>1</td></tr>
</table>

Figure 2: *Your levels of arousal and coping strategies help sheet.*

away. Maybe you're desperate to read more and more and see what the answer is. Whatever's there, whatever you're feeling or thinking, it's okay to just notice and recognise it for now. You don't have to do anything.

So, presuming you feel ready to start, let's go ahead and consider this more.

I invite you to ask yourself: why is it that this book is in your hands right now? What is it that has kept you from reading it until now?

There's something important here, behind these actions. There's something that's made you choose to take action on whatever's happening in your life right now and begin to explore it further. Perhaps it's a desire to be the best kind of parent you can be. Perhaps it's the hope that things can be different for your child than they were for you. Perhaps you want to give your child the kind of life where it's easy for them to find inner peace and happiness. Perhaps you're hoping to be able to support and care for somebody who's suffering.

Whatever the reason is, just see if you can connect with it right now, even if it's just a small kernel of a reason. Most importantly, begin by noticing what it is that you want to make this journey about: for you, for your baby, for your family, and broader still, for your world.

Stop. Notice what this is. Jot it down right here, right now.

MY INVITATION TO YOU

Throughout this section of the book, I'll invite you to take part in some exercises. It's really easy to want to just keep reading, without stopping to do the exercises. I know. I would be tempted to do the same thing! But I can tell you, having stopped and done the exercises myself, that you will gain so much more value than you would otherwise get from just reading. In fact, I think it will increase the potency of the book about a hundred times for you if you can pause and do the exercise each time.

So have a think and see if there is anything you would be willing to do to help make it more likely that you will take part in the exercises that are available for you here ...

Would you be willing to do them if it meant that you could become more like the parent that you most want to be? Would you be willing to do them if it meant that you could discover new and interesting things about yourself, even if they might be a little bit challenging? Or would you be willing to do it on the proviso that you can try them and see how it works for you? There'll be plenty of opportunities for you to stop and notice what's working for you and not working for you. So, I'd invite you to give the exercises a chance. Have a go, see how they work and then don't do any more if they're not helping you.

I'd invite you to make a commitment right now to do the exercises as they come up, and to not read any further until they're done. Go on. Try to link this internal commitment to your goals, to what you want this journey to do for you.

And just a reminder, this is always an invitation. You don't have to push yourself. It's not a demand. But if you decide not to do the exercises, I'd ask you to just observe what it's like. And then, if you can, try an exercise, and contrast the feeling to see which approach works for you.

WHY SO MANY METAPHORS?

Take a look at this picture opposite ...

Have you ever had this experience of your mind taking you for a walk, rather than the other way around? Think of those times when Sonya travelled to baby group, but didn't actually go inside. The part of her mind that told her it would be awkward

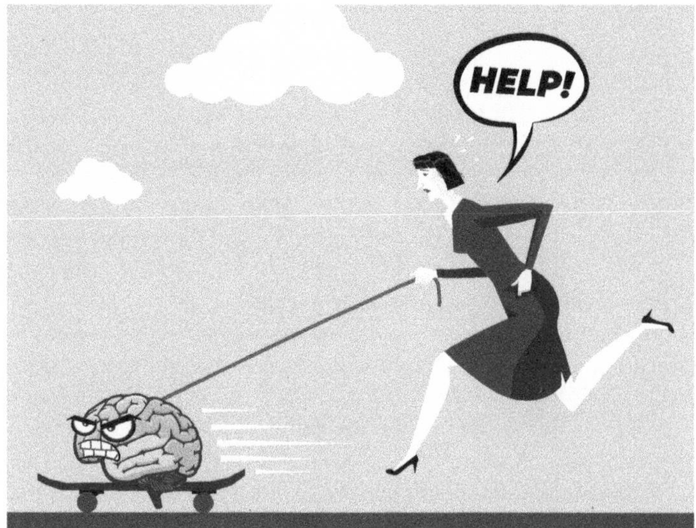

Figure 3: *Sometimes it feels like your mind is taking you for a walk.*

and embarrassing and difficult was taking her for a walk then, without her even realising it. This stopped her doing something that might actually have helped her.

How often does your subconscious mind decide what you do, rather than you choosing? This is the brilliant irony of therapy and of self-help books in general. It's quite possible that the language that we use to try to solve problems could be part of the problem in itself. Take a moment to consider this.

What if all of your thoughts, beliefs, wishes, dreams, memories, and hopes might be contributing in some way to the difficulties you're experiencing? That is why this book will have a lot of stories and a lot of metaphors; we're going to try to sneakily trick your mind so that you get to choose what happens. It's so that you can notice when your mind is being helpful. And you can choose to do something different if it's giving you solutions that are less helpful.

Don't get me wrong. Our minds are great at solving problems in the outside world. In the world outside of our skin, we're warm, we're dry, we're happy in a lot of ways because we have such awesome minds.

Often though, our minds are less useful for problems and struggles that are inside our skin: difficulties with thinking, feeling, and urges to do things.

The science that lies beneath an acceptance and commitment therapy approach suggests that language is a key part of the problem. We take it too seriously and we see it as real. So to help you get past your mind taking you for a walk, we're going to use metaphors to help you connect with your actual experiences. And besides, they're probably a lot more memorable than me explaining things to you endlessly anyway!

Throughout this book, I invite you to read what I say carefully, but don't feel like you need to believe everything I say at face value. Let's begin by throwing out the rule book. There we are – it's gone. There is no rule book with this journey you're going to take!

It's possible that you might have connected a little bit with this idea in your experience of becoming a mother. Sure, a rule book for motherhood might seem awesome, but actually, there are times when rules just get in the way of being able to learn from what's happening in the here and now.

So, rather than just believing what I say, always check back to see what your own experience told you. Notice what actually happened for you. Sometimes that's a little confusing. The good news is that, the more you practise it, the easier it will be to notice what actually happened – rather than what your mind told you had happened, or what I'm suggesting might have happened.

Let me give you an example. I come from a family where dummies (or pacifiers) are the "spawn of Satan!" You did not give a dummy to a baby in my family. Babies were born to suckle on nipples, and were breastfed.

When my son was born, he was desperate to suck. He wanted to suck on anything, and he wanted to suck all the time. Sucking actually helped him because he had terrible reflux and it allowed him to swallow more easily, which helped reduce his pain. We spent a very long time with our little fingers in our young son's mouth! He would suck and suck and suck, and eventually we realised that our fingers were probably covered with germs, and certainly a lot less convenient than using a dummy. We were operating under this rule that dummies were bad, and we had a baby who needed to suck. So we gave him a dummy. He didn't get distorted teeth, and he didn't have any problems with giving up the dummy when he was a little bit older. They were our fears. But his need was to suck. That's just one example of how functioning under a rule made it harder for me to do what worked.

So I invite you now to consider whether there are any rules that you are operating under that possibly get in the way of doing what works for you, your baby, and your family. Let's work together to get to a point where you do whatever it is that works for you in the long term.

NO MAGIC WANDS

Let me tell you some things that this book cannot do. Firstly, you'll notice that it's the wrong shape to be a magic wand. I'm not going to be able to help you get rid of all of your problems. Instead, I hope to help you perceive your life in new ways and find fresh perspectives on the fullness of life. I'll help you grasp the opportunity for your life to be bigger, more encompassing, more filled with growth, and curiosity, and openness. As a result, you can be more flexible and more available to the people you care about.

When you're ready to find out more, let's move on to the next section.

SECTION 3

WHERE DOES IT HURT?

START WITH ONE STRUGGLE ...

What's your struggle today? What's the thing that you find yourself fighting? What is it that you want to get rid of that's causing you more suffering? What is it that's present that's causing life to be unbearable.

Whatever it is, notice its presence as best as you can. See if you can find an object around you that could represent the feelings that you have about the struggle – something a bit like a monster. If you can't find an object, perhaps write it on paper, or on a computer, tablet, or phone screen in front of you.

Now I'd like you to clench your fists as tightly as you can – as if you were going to fight this thing. Feel that strong tension in your hands. Perhaps you feel that you'd like to physically punch this experience – to push it out of the way.

Continue to keep your hands really tight, and as you do this, notice how easy you think it would be to do something that you really care about right now, while you're in this state of wanting to fight this thing so much. How easy would it be to soothe your baby? How easy would it be to be curious and interested in a creative pursuit? How easy would it be to hug your partner?

Now, notice again the feeling of tension in your fingers and hands, and then let go. Observe the intensity of the difference in this feeling. Notice what it's like to just let go, and to not have to struggle so hard anymore. As you physically let go in your hands, see if you can psychologically let go of some of the fight you've been having with whatever difficult experience has been showing up for you.

Notice now, that whatever object or monster you attached to this experience is still there. It hasn't gone away or altered, and yet, right now, how much easier do you think it would be to do one of those things that really matter to you in your life? How much effort does it take to be present with what's hurting, compared to having to endure the hurt as well as the struggle?

This may be your first experience of doing just a little bit of letting go. As a famous TV shampoo ad once said, "It won't happen overnight, but it will happen". Letting go involves practise, practise, and more practise. And so, let's begin by looking at what it is you might want to use as the basis for making space and letting go.

WHAT ELSE ARE YOU STRUGGLING WITH?

As you do your Niagara-Falls-style balancing act of becoming a parent or supporting a parent, begin to expand your field of vision to notice all the things that you're struggling with. What are the parts that you've found hard? What causes you pain, and where does it hurt?

Begin by writing these things down. Sometimes you'll find it easy to sort these things into different categories. Other times, they'll seem amorphous, like that foggy cloud that can roll in above Niagara Falls. So, as best you can, observe the difficult thoughts that show up, the beliefs you have that cause you pain, and the emotions that you're struggling with. These might be emotions like sadness, anger, anxiety, frustration, and fear.

There might also be memories that are painful for you – maybe you have memories from the birth that are still difficult to deal with. Maybe your memories from childhood are showing up, or memories of times that it has been hard for you to connect with people.

There will be sensations in your body that accompany these things as well. What physical sensations hurt you or are painful? It might be butterflies in your stomach or the pounding of your heart when your baby wakes in the night. Maybe it's a leaden kind of sensation that accompanies feelings of sadness.

Finally, there's a category called urges to act. This one is a little bit difficult at first, but once you get your head around it, it's quite useful to notice. Urges to act are when you want to do something. It's the feeling that comes just before you do the thing you're thinking of.

For example, you might notice an urge to eat a treat, or an urge to race out of the room when you're stressed. It might even be an urge to do something that you know you'll never even act upon, like the urge to shake your baby, or scream at the top of your voice in a group of people.

If you can notice any of these things as they show up, jot them down too. It's really helpful for you to begin noticing these things. It's from this point on that noticing gives you the opportunity to make a choice about what you do when those urges show up, rather than being freaked out by them, or acting on them automatically.

Take your time and write it all down until you really feel like you've covered everything.

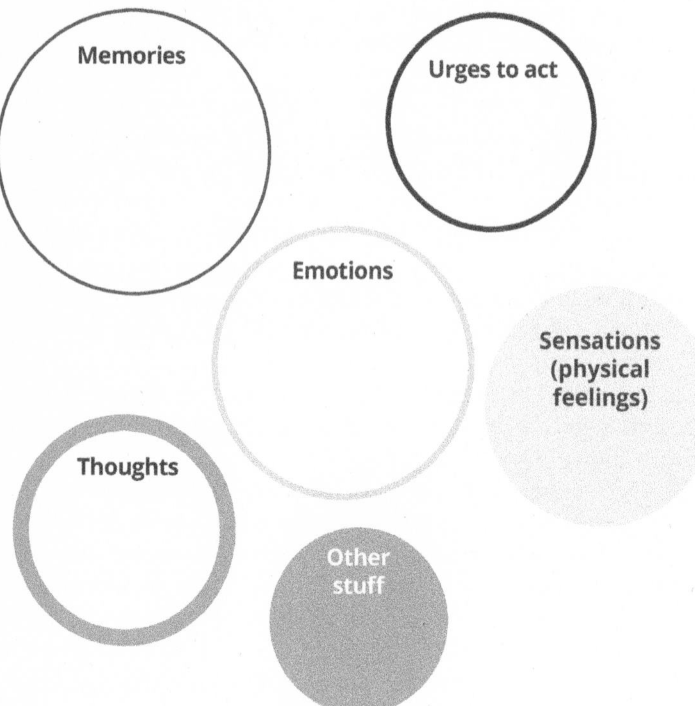

Figure 4: *Identify the difficult thoughts and painful emotions that show up for you.*

Here's an example, roughly based on Sonya's experience.

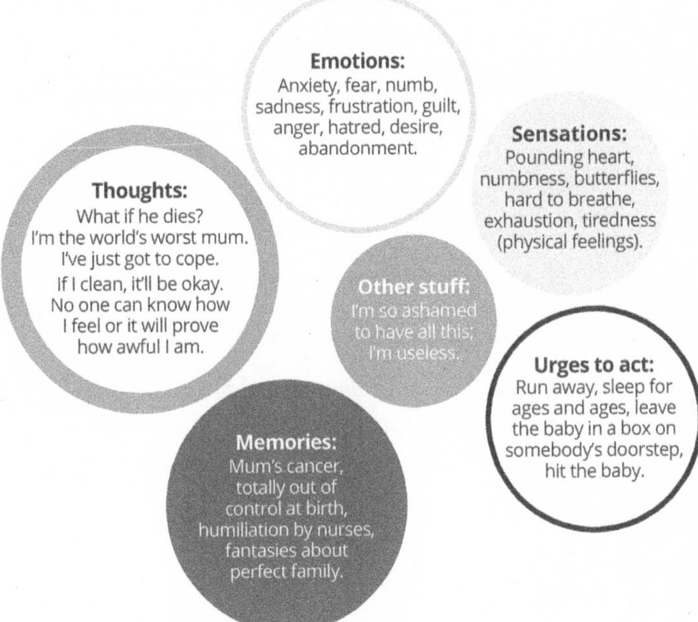
Emotions:
Anxiety, fear, numb, sadness, frustration, guilt, anger, hatred, desire, abandonment.
Sensations:
Pounding heart, numbness, butterflies, hard to breathe, exhaustion, tiredness (physical feelings).
Thoughts:
What if he dies?
I'm the world's worst mum.
I've just got to cope.
If I clean, it'll be okay.
No one can know how I feel or it will prove how awful I am.
Other stuff:
I'm so ashamed to have all this; I'm useless.
Urges to act:
Run away, sleep for ages and ages, leave the baby in a box on somebody's doorstep, hit the baby.
Memories:
Mum's cancer, totally out of control at birth, humiliation by nurses, fantasies about perfect family.

Figure 5: *Some of the difficult thoughts and painful emotions that showed up for Sonya.*

If there's not enough space, keep going on another sheet. Put it all on there. This is what hurts. I wish I could magic it away for you. No matter how hard I try (and believe me, I've tried!) the magic wand approach never works. Sometimes this pain is REALLY strong. It just is. Sometimes it's less intense than you realised. And very often it's what we do in response to this pain that can hurt us more: remember the difference between clenching your fists and letting go? The part you can make choices about, the part that is within your control (at least somewhat) is what you do when this pain manifests itself.

WHAT HAVE YOU DONE IN THE PAST WHEN THIS PAIN SHOWS UP?

Begin your list here. Don't worry about the two columns on either side – we'll get to those later. I've started you off with some examples – if they fit for you, feel free to use them! If not, just cross them out.

More of Same	What I've tried doing to cope or to fight against what hurts, or given up because of this hurt	Long Game
	Cleaned because it gives me feelings of control	
	Left the baby with someone else	
	Wished it would all go away and fantasised about the old days	

Next, take a moment to think, as you look at this page full of all the things that have been hurting you – all of the painful thoughts, memories, emotions, sensations, and urges to do things. Jot down anything that occurs to you to do, anything that you think can help you cope in some way. Even if it's the kind of thing that you think only helps in the long term rather than the short term.

To help you get a better idea of the difference between the things that are hurting you and what you're doing when that hurt or pain shows up, let's talk about another way of seeing this ...

Imagine you're standing blindfolded at the edge of a large field. You can feel the slightly squidgy sensation of the mud underneath the grass. You can smell the countryside smells.

You can't take your blindfold off, and you've been left here to find your own way back. You're carrying a fairly heavy bag. You step out gingerly, taking the first few steps, and then suddenly, find yourself falling. Bang! You're stuck in a deep hole. You can feel that the sides are straight and the hole is so deep that you start to feel really scared.

You think to yourself, *I'm holding onto this heavy bag. I wonder what's in it.* So you open it up and, using your hands, you feel some cold metal and a handle. You can make out the shape of a spade.

You're down the bottom of a hole and you have a spade. So what do you do? You dig. But hang on ... does digging help you get out of a hole? Notice what your mind does here. Minds can be very clever about working this out. For example, I've had people come up with the idea of digging steps up the side to get out.

Just take a moment to consider – when you're down at the bottom of a hole, is a spade what you really need? Or do you really need something else entirely?

I could give you a gold-plated spade. Would that be helpful? Or maybe a really powerful digger. Let's say I ship in with a helicopter and drop down to you with one of the most powerful diggers in the world ... but that's still not what you need right now ...

So in this scenario, what's the best thing to do?

Stop digging. Stop making the hole any deeper. Just because you've been given a spade, you don't have to use it.

Although you didn't know it, this field was full of holes. It's not your fault that the field is full of holes. But you would have landed in one sooner or later. And you would have instinctively begun using the tool you were given. Be kind to yourself about this.

In this metaphor, the field is life. We all head out blindly into life and, sooner or later, we all encounter something that, by its very nature, causes us pain or is difficult. So we use our mind – that works so well for us in so many other scenarios – to help us solve things. It's like the spade. I could work with you to give you a much, much better set of things to do with your mind to fight this stuff that shows up and hurts so much.

I'm not going to, though.

Because, like digging when you're down a hole, I don't believe it's helpful. And it's not just me. There's actually really good research that suggests that using the thing that got you into this mess (your mind, your language) is probably not the thing that is going to be most helpful at getting you out.

So, great news – you've begun to notice this stuff. You're noticing what you've done to struggle, what you've fought against, and what you've given up in order to cope.

So what are the ways that you have tried to dig yourself out of the difficulties of looking after your baby? Here are some examples to get you going. Have you:

Stayed in bed?

Handed the baby over to somebody else?

Wished it would all go away?

Fantasised about the old days?

Tried to do everything perfectly?

You know, some of the things that you've done in response to the painful stuff have probably been helpful for you in the long term. So don't beat yourself up about this.

Unfortunately, as human beings, we're really well programmed to want to do things that are immediately helpful, that immediately take away painful feelings and make us feel better. Or even make us try to numb or forget the pain.

In the real world, this kind of approach works beautifully. In the real world, if I buy a pair of boots that I decide are a bit of a mistake, I can stick them in the back of my wardrobe and never have to think about them. Well, at least until I tidy my wardrobe, when I might decide to get rid of them. But you can't do this with difficult feelings.

If those boots had actually been self-doubt and feelings of being a terrible mother, then I could try sticking them at the back of my mind. But inside your skin, this rule doesn't work so well (even if your mind keeps trying to make it work!) Unlike the boots, the pain of self-doubt and guilt will just keep rising to the surface. If guilt and self-doubt were boots in a wardrobe, it would be like they have a life of their own and keep wiggling to the front of the wardrobe, jumping onto our feet as soon as we opened the door.

Check in with your own experience and see if this is true for you as well. When you've tried to get rid of something inside of you, how has it worked out for you in the long term? Has it gone away for good? Or has it come back later, bringing more of the same, and taking you away from what really matters?

I invite you now to get a couple of coloured pens and work through the list that you wrote. In one colour, highlight the things that might have worked and felt really good in the short term. That's why you do those things, of course. With the other pen, highlight what worked well in the long term.

What helped you move towards the things that matter most?

The things that will work well in the long term will sometimes work all right in the short term. But sometimes you'll find that they're really quite painful in the short term.

An example from my own life is training to go uphill on my bike. I love mountain biking, but it takes quite a lot of pain when I have to do the hard yards to get up the hill. And yet I know that, in the long term, it's something that massively enriches my life.

So again, it's not your fault that you haven't done this stuff. We're made as humans to rail against going through the hard stuff first before we get to the good parts later on. But the cool part is that you can use your knowledge and your awareness to help you begin to recognise the things that work better in the long term. And, you can plot your course to help take you in that direction.

Here's another way of thinking about this: it's a bit like when you have a car that you keep patching up because you can't afford to buy a new one. So you keep doing short-term fixes until one day, bang! Your car experiences a terminal event. You absolutely have to buy another car. Will you have saved enough money to at least buy one that needs fewer band-aid fixes?

Noticing what you're doing in response to your pain is a little bit like that process of saving up. It's like building a stronger, more easily able-to-respond version of you. One that's more flexible, and doesn't need so many short-term fixes.

If you begin to do what works in the longer term, you might find that there are fewer breakdowns along the way.

This is what I'm talking about when I say, 'How does that work?' I'm asking: how does that work in the long term? How does it work, long-term, to do band-aid fixes? How has it worked when you've done things that help in the long run?

Think of this as playing the long game rather than resorting to more of the same coping strategies. Now return to your list, and draw arrows to show which of your strategies have taken you in either direction. Be careful here! Sometimes strategies that seem like long-term measures can sneakily be more of your usual quick-fix mechanisms.

Sometimes there might be an element of a "more of the same" strategy mixed in with a long game element. In that scenario, see if you can tease it apart a bit more. What is the part of your coping strategy that works in the long run?

To be clear here, it's your own experience that matters. You may find that what's a serious more-of-the-same move for someone else actually contributes to your long game. For example, leaving the baby with someone else could be one way to have a bit of both. When Sonya and Devon gave themselves a break overnight by leaving Jack with someone, it gave them some desperately needed rest, which in turn may have allowed them space to make clearer choices about how to cope long-term. For another person, repeatedly handing their baby over to someone else can become a pattern which doesn't fix anything for the future. In time, the parent may feel less and less competent with their own baby and become increasingly anxious about caring for them. Perhaps it'll get to the point where they will avoid doing as much of the care as they can.

You need to check your own experience here, rather than comparing it to others or just taking my word for it.

You are not alone in your pain. Nor are you alone in having unwittingly done things that don't work very well and may unfortunately amplify what hurts. That is part of being human. I suspect you never had the chance to notice that those more-of-the-same coping strategies were actually building a bigger and bigger mountain of pain. Not only are our brains set up this way, but our societies are set up to encourage us to do what works short-term too. Think of all the advertising that suggests that, if you just buy a particular product, you'll finally get happiness, or get rid of what you don't want. Fast!

You came by your pain honestly. And you are not alone. In the next section, we'll see just how not alone you really are.

SECTION 4

WHAT IS THIS ABOUT? SOME INFORMATION ABOUT PERINATAL MENTAL HEALTH

"Perinatal mental illness remains a leading cause of maternal death (Knight et al., 2014) with over half of women who tragically die during this time having a previous history of severe mental illness and half of deaths caused by suicide."

(Perinatal Mental Health Alliance 2015).

The year after having a baby, a woman is more at risk of becoming mentally unwell than at any other time in her entire life. The term "perinatal" means "around childbirth". Frequently, all mental illness in the perinatal period is put under the umbrella term of postnatal depression. My preference is to use the term perinatal, as it fits better with the facts, and reminds us that often mental illness starts prior to, or during pregnancy, for both men and women.

What is depression? Sonya's story illustrates many of the characteristics clinicians use to diagnose depression: tearfulness, misery, lack of enjoyment, lack of motivation, lack of sexual interest, and wanting to die / planning for suicide. We often look for disruptions in sleep and appetite as well, either too much or too little of either. The criteria for ante- and postnatal depression are the same as depression at any other point. As you can imagine, sleep is not such a helpful indicator during pregnancy or postnatally, so we often look at this somewhat differently: how hard is it to get to sleep when you get the chance (if you do)? What is it that stops you from eating or sleeping?

Another aspect is duration and frequency of these symptoms: for a diagnosis of a depressive episode, a duration of at least two weeks – with symptoms present for a longer amount of time than they are not – required.

The Edinburgh Postnatal Depression Scale (Cox, Holden and Sagovsky, 1987) is a good screening tool to see if you're at risk of depression or anxiety after childbirth. Scores of 13 or more suggest you're at risk.

Edinburgh Postnatal Depression Scale (EPDS)

J.L. Cox, J.M. Holden, R. Sagovsky; Department of Psychiatry, University of Edinburgh

How are you feeling?

Your Name:

Date Today:

As you have recently had a baby, we would like to know how you are feeling. Please UNDERLINE the answer which comes closest to how you have felt IN THE PAST 7 DAYS, not just how you feel today.

Here is an example, already completed.
I have felt happy:
Yes, all the time | Yes, most of the time
No, not very often | No, not at all

This would mean "I have felt happy most of the time during the past week." Please complete the other questions in the same way.

IN THE PAST 7 DAYS:

1. I have been able to laugh and see the funny side of things:
As much as I always could | Not quite so much now
Definitely not so much now | No not at all

2. I have looked forward with enjoyment to things:
As much as I ever did | Rather less than I used to
Definitely less than I used to | Hardly at all

***3. I have blamed myself unnecessarily when things went wrong:**
Yes, most of the time | Not very often
Yes, some of the time | No, never

4. I have been anxious or worried for no good reason:
No, not at all | Hardly ever
Yes, sometimes | Yes, very often

Figure 6: *The Edinburgh Postnatal Depression Scale (EPDS).*

Edinburgh Postnatal Depression Scale (EPDS)

J.L. Cox, J.M. Holden, R. Sagovsky; Department of Psychiatry, University of Edinburgh

IN THE PAST 7 DAYS (continued):

5. I have felt scared and panicky for no good reason:

Yes, quite a lot	Yes, sometimes
No, not much	No, not at all

6. Things have been getting on top of me:

Yes, most of the time I haven't been able to cope at all

Yes, sometimes I haven't been coping as well as usual

No, most of the time I have been coping quite well

No, I have been coping as well as ever

7. I have been so unhappy I've had difficulty sleeping:

Yes, most of the time	Yes, quite often
Not very often	No, not at all

8. I have felt sad or miserable:

Yes, most of the time	Yes, quite often
Only occasionally	No, never

9. I have been so unhappy that I have been crying:

Yes, most of the time	Yes, quite often
Only occasionally	No, never

10. The thought of harming myself has occurred to me:

Yes, quite often	Sometimes
Hardly ever	Never

Answer Key:

For items 1, 2 & 4

0	1
2	3

For all other items

3

2

1

Figure 6: *The Edinburgh Postnatal Depression Scale (EPDS).*

This mix of depression and anxiety was evident for Sonya. It was present in her description of her drive to clean, which soothed her anxiety and worry. In my practice, I frequently meet mothers who experience symptoms of obsessive compulsive disorder (OCD), panic, or generalised anxiety disorder alongside their depression. Sometimes this is severe enough to meet a diagnosis for one or more anxiety disorders as well.

What can severe anxiety look like? Here are some brief descriptions of the most common kinds of anxiety in the postpartum, with the aim of helping you recognise whether you might be experiencing a specific kind of anxiety (although an actual diagnosis would need more than just the symptoms I describe here).

OCD involves thoughts which are hard to escape from, often around themes of harm, contagion, or need for order and control (obsessions). In turn, people experiencing OCD will often do some kind of routine or ritual to neutralise these thoughts or fears. That's the compulsion.

Panic attacks are a sudden, massive rush of anxiety or sense of overwhelm, with particular physical symptoms like a racing heart, fast breathing, dizziness, shaking, sweating, and often a strong urge to escape. Sometimes people can think they are having a heart attack or going crazy when they panic, which naturally makes them even more terrified. The good news is that no one has ever died from a panic attack, and there are lots of options for treatment.

Generalised anxiety disorder (GAD) involves constant worry, sometimes centred on several particular themes, sometimes floating from one target to another. People with GAD often describe themselves as "born worriers", and worry can end up being perceived as necessary in order to solve problems or to help them stay safe from potential harm. This can then result in a vicious cycle of self-perpetuating worry, reassurance-seeking and inaction.

Like most people, clinicians come in "lumpers" or "splitters". I am a lumper: I tend to see the anxiety and depression as often functionally related to one another, and look to treat what I formulate as the common underlying issues there.

Research suggests that experiential avoidance may underlie a wide range of psychopathology (Hayes, Strosahl and Wilson, 2012). Experiential avoidance is just a big name for doing, or not doing, lots of things, so as to not have to experience difficult emotions, thoughts, sensations, memories or urges to do something. Sometimes we're well aware of choosing to do or not do things. Other times it's such a long-established pattern or something that's begun so early in life that we're not even aware we're doing it anymore.

For example, Sonya's cleaning meant she didn't have to be present with the immense loss of control she had in her life. It immediately gave her a sense of potency and achievement when she had few other opportunities to experience this. In the short term, she cleaned and felt better. All humans do things that make us feel better straight away, it's how we're designed! Unfortunately, this is also a great cause of suffering: what works in the short term may or may not work well in the long term. As Sonya observes, her cleaning became increasingly obsessive, as she used it more and more for the quick hit of control it gave her. Soon enough, the cleaning itself became another source of suffering, linking into fears about how others would evaluate her and stopping her from being able to do things she might enjoy. Working with the exercises in the second half of this book is very likely to help you increase your psychological flexibility.

So how is the splitter perspective useful?

It is useful in helping us pull apart types of symptoms and their severity, to consider how widespread particular problems are. It's also helpful when it comes to rarer conditions like bipolar disorder and psychosis, as these need quite different kinds of treatment. If you have previously been diagnosed with bipolar disorder or psychosis, it is important to seek consultation with a specialist perinatal service as soon as possible.

Ideally this ought to happen before you even conceive (NICE, 2014), but any time is better than waiting. Around 1-in-1000 women will experience psychosis after giving birth. Psychosis is the experience of hearing, seeing, or feeling things that aren't actually there, or having firm, fixed and unusual beliefs that don't have a strong basis in reality. Psychosis associated with bipolar disorder is known as mania, and involves a period of several days with symptoms such as feelings of expansive happiness, extremely high levels of activity, and extreme impulsivity which are out of character for the person's usual behaviour.

The highest risk time for psychosis to appear is soon after birth, and there is some suggestion that the interruption of sleep / wake cycles around labour - combined with the massive stress and change - may trigger the illness for a small percentage of women. If you have a close relative who has had bipolar disorder, psychosis, or schizophrenia, please discuss this with your health care team, as you are at higher risk in this case. Although, please do remember that the actual risk is still very low.

You are not alone

- 10–15% of women experience postpartum depression (Swain et al, 1997; Bledsoe and Grote, 2006).
- 10% of men experience postpartum depression (Paulson and Bazemore, 2010).
- Of women with postpartum depression, roughly one third are depressed prior to pregnancy. Another third become depressed during pregnancy, and the final third become depressed after the baby is born (Wisner, Sit and McShea et al, 2013).
- Around 20% of women with postpartum depression think about harming themselves. (Wisner et al, 2013).
- Two thirds of women with postpartum depression also have an anxiety disorder.

The risks are useful to know about

It's helpful to know what risk factors there are for experiencing perinatal mental illness, as then you have the power to make choices that can help minimise your risk (as Sonya did the second time around).

According to a systematic review by Biaggi et al. (2016), general risk factors for depression and anxiety include:

- Lack of partner or social support
- History of abuse or domestic violence
- Personal history of mental illness
- Unplanned or unwanted pregnancy

- Adverse events in life and high levels of perceived stress
- Present / past pregnancy complications
- Miscarriage

If you've had postpartum depression in the past, your risk for getting it again is around 25% (Robertson et al, 2004).

It's also important to know that there are very real risks associated with not treating mental health problems during pregnancy. It is painful to know that if you've been depressed during pregnancy, this is likely to have had an impact upon your baby. Remember, though, that having this knowledge allows you to make choices to help your child from this point onwards. Again, it speaks to the importance of getting help as soon as possible in the future.

- Anxiety and depression in pregnancy are strongly associated with adverse outcomes for mothers and babies including preterm birth and low birth weight (Dunkel-Schetter 2011; Dunkel-Schetter and Tanner 2012).
- Children of depressed mothers are more likely to suffer depression themselves (Ashman and Dawson, 2012).
- Maternal depression and anxiety affect the developing foetus via cortisol levels, which has a lifelong effect upon the child's ability to regulate their emotions (Bergener, Monk and Werner, 2008).
- Depression in the father during the postnatal period is also associated with adverse emotional and behavioural outcomes in children aged three–five years (Ramchandari et al, 2008).
- Maternal depression has been shown in a large meta-analysis to increase the likelihood of both disorganised and insecure attachment styles, and significantly reduce the likelihood of secure attachment styles (Martins and Gaffan, 2000).

Notice that these connections are not deterministic: a mother's depression and anxiety will not inevitably lead to interruptions in her relationship with her baby or future negative consequences for her baby's health, although it does raise the chance of this happening.

Things can be done to help

- Women often recover within a few months.
- Receiving a psychosocial or psychological intervention significantly reduces the risk of women developing depression in the first place (Dennis and Dowswell, 2013).
- Psychological interventions (e.g. Cognitive Behavioural Therapy, interpersonal therapy) help women get better sooner (JAMA, 2016) although the evidence is somewhat mixed about whether this is better than standard care according to meta-analysis (Perveen et al., 2013).
- Cognitive Behavioural Therapy (CBT) prevention and intervention lowers rates of postpartum depression compared to standard care (Sockol, 2015).
- Compared to placebos, antidepressant medication (selective serotonin reuptake inhibitors or SSRI types) show better response and higher remission rates for postpartum depression (Molyneux, Trevillion and Howard, 2015). This may be an underestimation, as women with severe depression or suicidal ideation are seldom included in such studies. There are some concerns regarding the safety of anti-depressants for pregnant and breastfeeding mothers (Yonkers et al., 2014).
- SSRI medication and psychotherapy perform roughly equally in effectiveness in randomised controlled trials (O'Hara and McCabe, 2013).
- Other psychological interventions also show promise according to trials, including compassion-focused therapy, mindfulness interventions, and parent-infant dyadic therapy.

Important things for society to address

- Recognition and treatment rates for depression are even lower in pregnant and postpartum women (14%) than in the general population (26%) (Bennett et al., 2010).
- Suicide was the most common cause of perinatal maternal death in New Zealand from 2006 – 2013 (PMMRC, 2015).
- The average cost to society of one case of perinatal depression is around £74,000 in the UK (Baur et al., 2014).

- Maternal prepartum anxiety and depression alone may account for up to 10–15% of negative emotional and behavioural outcomes in children's lives (Glover, 2014).

Seeking help for yourself, supporting your loved ones and friends in getting help, and using this book are all things that will protect you in the longer term. For Sonya and me, this is what Pulling the Trigger is actually about: pulling the trigger on the floodgates of change around parenting and mental illness in our society. Identification and treatment of peripartum mental illness is an important social and economic issue, in terms of saving lives, saving money and improving outcomes for the next generation.

Attachment and bonding

At some level, all of us have had an experience of babies. After all, we were all babies once upon a time! The difficult part is that our memories from this time aren't verbal memories. There aren't any words, or even images, that we can call up and remember.

Psychologists call these kinds of memories implicit or nondeclarative memories. These are just fancy terms for memories that are formed of feelings and sensations of touch, smell, sounds, and a sense of safety and contentment or fear and disconnection. Because they're not related to words, it's a real challenge for us as adults to realise that these things are even memories. They are probably seen as facts that we know about the world, e.g. the sense that the world is a safe place, or the sense that, if you're distressed, no one really cares. These things come through the process of our own attachment relationships with our parents. The beauty of the attachment relationship is that it has probably allowed our species to survive and thrive in a way we might not otherwise have done. Human babies are born incredibly vulnerable compared to almost every other kind of species. They have big heads, they can't walk or talk, and they can barely communicate their needs in a way that adults find easy to understand.

The intense bonding that can happen – and often does happen – at the very first stages of a child's life helps keep the parents around long enough to care for their child. This way the child can become bigger, stronger, and more likely to survive. The beauty of this is that the parent gradually learns the non-verbal language that the baby uses in order to communicate with them. The pain of this is that the memories of our own childhood are non-verbal and are created in relationship to another human being.

Because we're often unaware that these are even memories, these patterns in relationships tend to elicit very old behaviour that we're unaware of. And because we're unaware of them, they're very hard to change, precisely because these patterns are not part of our verbal system.

At the same time, that's the beauty of our own attachment memory. Being in this relationship with your baby is an opportunity to discover where you got your own sense of safety or fear for the world. It helps you find out what you need in the world and in a relationship (if that's not something you've had the chance to find out before.) You can try new things, learn to connect in new ways and see some different perspectives.

This is the great challenge, though: why would you want to try something new when you're terrified for your life? Remember that idea of setting off on a rope over Niagara Falls?

If you're swamped by challenging history from your past, or you've never had a chance to learn to meet your own needs, if you know nothing about babies or you haven't had the opportunity to bond with your baby early on, it's really hard work. And it's really bad luck.

I have a hypothesis about why bonding is sometimes delayed. In the past, babies died. Lots. Mothers died a lot too. Many traditional societies didn't actually accept babies into the tribe until they were between three and twelve months old. If, as a mother, you immediately experienced a really strong bond, you risked having your heart broken repeatedly.

Personally, I think it's a myth that we fall head over heels in love every time with every child. Think about the love that you've had (and that you have right now) for many different people in your life. Is that love the same every time and in every way? Sometimes love can be slow, sometimes fast. Sometimes sudden, sometimes gradual. Sometimes soft, sometimes intense. Sometimes it's easy to do; sometimes it's much more challenging.

Why would it be any different with a baby? Add on to this all the factors we've discussed already: the expectations you've had, the interruptions that have happened, the massive social change, and lack of support. It begins to explain why it can be so hard for us as parents sometimes to connect with our babies.

But as Sonya's story shows, it doesn't mean it can't happen.

Allow yourself some space and some time for it to begin happening for you. Hold yourself gently as you start to notice some of the things that could be helpful for you in this journey.

SECTION 5

FINDING A DIRECTION TO GO

Let's take a moment to think about what matters most ...

We can spend a lot of time in our lives desperately trying to get away from things that are painful for us, or make life harder for us. There's an alternative to this – and perhaps you've noticed it already. It's orienting yourself towards what matters and slowly, step by step, going in that direction.

This is a little bit like how people used to navigate once upon a time, using the sun. By working out when the sun rose, roughly what direction east was, and when the sun set, you'd know aspects of your environment that would help you remember where west was. The sun can help to orient us and it's not a fixed destination.

What matters most to us – our values, in other words – are often not like goals. In fact, they're the precise opposite of goals: they're not sensible, measurable, achievable, realistic, or time-limited. If you can think of things that are the opposite of smart goals, then you're probably well on your way to working out what a value is.

Let's say the direction I choose to go in is west. I start from my home and eventually I'll hit my workplace. And then I'll go across the plains, and I'll know I'm going west when I hit the mountains. And then, once I get over the mountains, I'll hit the west coast of the South Island. And that'll tell me that I've gone a good way west.

Now, if I'm ready to get my feet wet, I can keep going. And if I'm willing to get wet all over, I can keep going west until I hit Melbourne or Adelaide. And I don't even have to stop there. I can keep on going west and get really very, very wet and keep going all the way to South America. I can keep going west as long as I want to, just going round and round the world.

Learning to do what matters most to you, and moving forward in that direction, is a bit like that kind of journey.

Let's take a moment for you to begin to orient yourself towards what matters for you. Given that you're reading a book that's related to parenting, I suggest we begin by considering what matters most to you about being a parent – by exploring what you would most like your child to receive from the experience of having you as a parent.

Let's look forward a few years – imagine your son or daughter is having a huge twenty-first birthday party, and during the party, they speak to everyone about what they most valued about you as their parent. It doesn't matter if your child hasn't even been conceived yet, you can still give it a go. (This exercise is based on the Funeral Exercise by Hayes, Wilson and Strosahl, 2012.)

Think about what you would most like to hear your child say about the things that you'd done for them, and the ways in which you'd supported them. You can make this entirely self-focused, and you don't need to worry whether it's a realistic vision of what a "typical" twenty-one-year-old might say!

In a moment, I'm going to ask you to set the book aside and find a comfortable space so that you can bring to mind where the birthday party might take place. Perhaps it's in a grand hall, or at somebody's house. Maybe it's outside in a park or garden. Really try to imagine yourself into this space – imagine what you can see, what you can hear, and what you can feel around you. Go a step further and try to imagine the taste of the birthday cake.

The more of your senses you engage, the better. And, because it's your imagination, you can have anybody you like attending the party. So, go and do this now and listen to what you would most like to hear your child say about how you parented them, and what mattered to them about the kind of parent you were. Focus on hearing what you would most like to hear your child say, not what they might actually say.

Done it? If you haven't, go back and give it a go.

Okay, now jot down some little things that you want to remember about what you've imagined. Perhaps there were things that you already knew about yourself. Or maybe there were some surprises in there. What matters so much to you about how you do this parenting job that you desperately want your child to talk about it when they turn twenty-one?

One of the coolest things about values is that you totally get to choose them yourself. No one else can dictate to you what your values are.

Your values might be so strong that you would still uphold them even if you were the last person left standing on earth. Of course, it would be difficult to hold values about relationships if there was nobody to have any kind of a relationship with. But humour me here! Look at those things you have written down, the things that you would still care about, even if no one else could know what you cared about so deeply. That shows just how important they are to you – and to your sense of being a good person and a good mother.

Some of the values that the mothers that I've worked with have talked about include love, connectedness, consistency (i.e. "Mum was always there for me"), curiosity, playfulness, fun, joy, boundaries, morality. These are just some examples. If any of them struck a chord with you, feel free to add them in as well.

Now let's look at moving a little bit beyond parenting and moving into thinking about the other areas of your life that you care about. To do this we're going to use this illustration of the sun, because I think about values as a bit like an awesome sunset behind the mountains. It ties in with what I said earlier about going west. Imagine that the rays of the sun are your values and the different areas of your life that really matter to you. Often these areas that we value change over time.

One of the biggest things about becoming a parent is that the relative weight and importance that we place on these values changes quite often and dramatically. Becoming a parent can move relationship values into focus that you possibly didn't even know were there. You can have new opportunities and challenges around boundaries, and newer opportunities to connect with people that you thought you'd never wish to connect with ever again. It can often mean that values around learning or employment fade a little. Some people find that becoming a parent helps them feel more connected with their spirituality.

Begin to think about the different areas on the sun diagram and jot down some of the things that you care about in each of these areas. You'll probably find that there are some that go across a number of them, and that's cool.

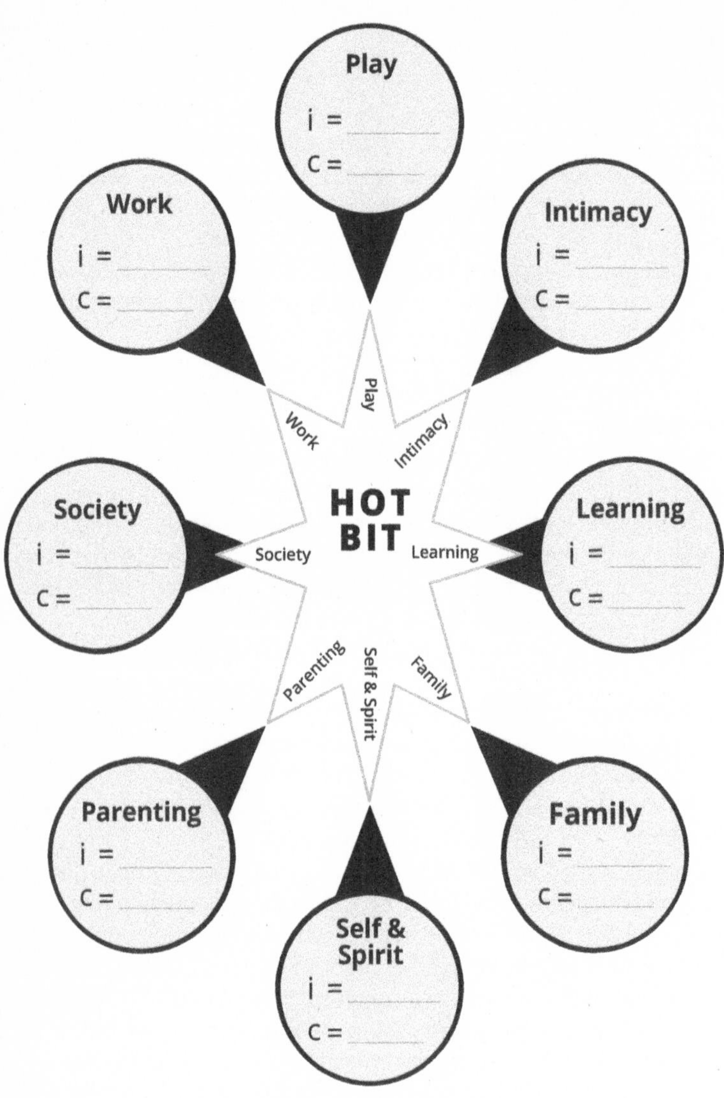

Figure 7: *Sun diagram based on the values compass created by JoAnne Dahl and Tobias Lundgren (2006).*

As you go through and start to look at all these things, it wouldn't be at all surprising if some painful feelings, sensations, emotions, or thoughts emerge. There's a really good reason for that. In the same way that the sun is hot, and its rays burn us, sometimes when we start thinking about the things that matter most to us, it feels a bit like we're going to get hurt. After all, things can only hurt us if they really matter to us, and it's the things we care about the most that cause us the most pain. These things are two sides of the same coin.

As you begin to recognise your values, notice also when any sore spots show up, and jot them down in the centre of the sun. Perhaps it hurts to think about trust and your relationship with your child, when your own trust has been betrayed so badly in the past. Maybe as you start to notice the things that you desperately cared about in your employment or in your learning in the past, it'll hurt because you feel disconnected from that right now, or because that part of you is less important at this moment. As best you can, be kind with yourself about this. Notice what's hurting, write it down and then notice any of the judgements that are coming up as you do that.

For example, your mind tells you that if you were a better person you would've learnt more and known more about being a parent. Or perhaps it will ask you how you can love this baby when no one has ever really loved you. Maybe there's heartache or sorrow in there, or maybe there's joy. Whatever's in there, see if you can just allow it to be there for now and gently and kindly bring your focus back to noticing what it is you care about, noticing any barriers or hotspots that come up as you do it.

What did you discover filling in this diagram?

You're not actually finished yet. The next task is to go back and think about how important each of these areas are in your life, at this point in time, and at this current moment. And again, this is totally about you and about what *you* feel about this.

You might be thinking, *I should feel like being a parent is absolutely the most important thing in my world right now.* But that might not actually be how it is for you. It's okay to rate it as high or low as it feels for you. Use a scale of 0 to 10, 0 being "It's not important at all", and 10 being "This is incredibly important".

You can add multiple 10s and multiple 0s if you want. Fill this in beside the "i=__" at the base of each box.

Okay, narrow it down again, and this time I'll ask you to note down how consistently you're putting this value into play in this area at the moment.

Let me explain a little bit more about this, because this is a bit of a tricky concept. How consistently are you acting on these values in this area of your life? Say your values for self-care were health, sustainability, fun, and compassion. Could you say that everything you do, and the way that you take care of yourself, takes you in the direction of these values? Can you say that you are 100% consistent with it? If that's the case, then your consistency would be a 10.

If you're less consistent - maybe you only work towards that value some of the time - it might be that your consistency is a 5. Or, if you're busy beating yourself up all the time and you don't put yourself first - if it's really hard for you to take any care of yourself, and consequently you find yourself feeling overwhelmed quite frequently - that might suggest that consistency score is 0, or perhaps a 1. Go ahead and do these ratings for the "c=___" space in each box.

As you do this exercise, you're probably going to need to make room for that pain - that heat from the sunrays burning you again. This is the kind of pain that can stop us from going towards what we really care about. We can often turn away and see it as a sign that we're pushing into something we don't want to go towards. But what if this heat was actually a sign you're on the right path, and that you're going towards what matters? What kind of difference would that make for you if it were the case? What do you think it would mean about how you might grow and develop as a person?

You might have begun to observe that babies grow so fast, but that their growth rarely comes without an accompanying pain. One example of this is teething. It hurts to grow teeth, it's painful, it gives the baby fevers, makes them dribble everywhere, and makes them wake up in the night because it hurts. The baby doesn't know it's for a greater good, but one day they'll be able to start eating solids and enjoy a wider range of foods. It will even help them move towards independence from their mother and their parents who have fed them to this point – but it's still not an easy thing to do. Sometimes, going towards what matters is rather like teething. It's hard to do in the short term and yet incredibly productive and helpful in the longer term. So, as best you can, be gentle and kind with yourself about the pain that emerges as you do this exercise.

Okay, this is the last part. I'd like you to look around that sun and consider for yourself where the biggest differences are between importance of a value and the consistency with which you work towards it.

So, for example, if you have been engaging with the community as a 7 / 10 and yet you're a 1 / 10 on how consistently you do it, then that shows a bit of a discrepancy. That probably means that it causes you a bit of pain because you're not doing what you want to do and what matters most to you.

It's understandable that you haven't had the time or energy to dedicate to achieving this goal. You may well have been in survival mode for a long time, and at the moment you might be much more committed to doing the things you need to do for your family. However, that also suggests that this part of your life isn't going the way you want it to.

Begin to see if you can think of some very, very small steps that you're not currently doing, but you could do, to take you in the direction of the things that matter to you. Would you be willing to set aside ten minutes a day to do that thing? Could you do it in combination with something else you're already doing? Could you link it to something you do regularly to remind you to do it?

Write down a step or action that you're not currently doing that will take you in the direction of one of your values. Make it little. Make it so that you can be pretty confident that you're going to go ahead and do it.

My step is ....

....

Try giving yourself a timeframe, and if you're really brave, tell other people that you're intending to do this. There's nothing that makes you go through with a commitment like telling other people.

I'll do this ....

....

And when you do this thing, rate it for yourself from your experience of it. Did it make you feel more connected with the things that you cared about? Did you feel like you were going in the direction that you wanted to go in?

After doing this step, I am ....

....

If the answer is yes, you felt more connected, keep going. If no, go back to the drawing board. There is more help with this later in the book. Try something else – see if you can find some things that help you grow *with* the pain, rather take you away from it.

SECTION 6

MAKING SPACE: WILLINGNESS AND ACCEPTANCE

Sonya's story is so painful in part because it illustrates how factors beyond our control can affect our lives. Psychologists are usually quite good at helping people make change in areas that are within the realm of their own control. The difficulty comes when life serves up bitter lemons, and there are few opportunities to make lemonade. In this scenario, humans often respond with hopelessness, or end up blaming themselves in a desperate attempt to get some sense of control back (even if it makes them the baddy). But, there is another option here. I'm going to illustrate it rather than explain it, because it's a subtle thing and can be hard to get your head around ...

Norma, the annoying neighbour at your party (a metaphor about willingness and commitment)

Imagine you've moved into the perfect neighbourhood. You've moved into your dream house in the place you've always wanted to live. Perhaps it's a cottage, a mansion, or a stunning new apartment. You're so excited to move in and meet your great new neighbours. To celebrate, you throw a housewarming party, and invite utterly everyone in the neighbourhood. You're desperate to meet all the other awesome people who live in your new area. You even go as far as putting up notices on the lampposts!

It's the day of the party. The lawns are freshly mown, you can smell the savouries baking in the oven, and there are trays of drinks ready for the taking. Your guests begin to arrive, and with them, happy thoughts about the new friends you'll make in this neighbourhood. You stand on the doorstep, welcoming them in, greeting each guest in turn. The party gets into swing, the music starts playing, there's the sound of chatter all around.

Then ... Norma turns up. You've seen her from a distance before now, and marvelled at how unfriendly she seems. You've observed other people get that trapped look around her, appearing like they're desperate to escape her clutches. She speaks. Her voice is grating, absurd. Nearly fainting from the overwhelming wafts of her perfume, you get that sinking feeling: *Here goes my party, here goes any hope I've had of fitting into my new neighbourhood*. Naturally, you decide you've got to stop her ruining your party. You'll send her to the kitchen and reduce the impact of her presence. But Norma's highly sociable, she's not easily sent away, and she re-captures your attention.

'Why won't you let me out? Is this actually MY surprise birthday party? Ooh, goodie, did I tell you about the time ...'

Every time you get into a good conversation with another guest, you spot Norma leaving the kitchen and furiously depart to herd her away from more of your guests. You herd her back into the kitchen. Norma gets increasingly annoyed and begins objecting loudly:

'What kind of party is this?! I haven't even finished my drink! Why do you want to get rid of me? Ooh, hello Penelope and David, let me introduce ...'

And there you are, shame-facedly meeting your lovely new neighbours in the company of Norma. What will they think of you? What's more, there are so many other people you'd like to meet, and time is passing quickly.

What kind of party is this for you? How can you enjoy it while you're constantly keeping track of Norma? Before you know it, it's getting late, you've had a dozen interrupted conversations, and your neighbours are beginning to glower at you. Do you really want to spend your party like this?

So, what can you do here? After all, you did invite everyone. Diverting, hiding and trying to get rid of Norma really hasn't worked, and meanwhile you're missing all the good bits.

Any ideas of what you could do?

What would it be like to welcome Norma in, even if you don't like her? Have you done anything like this before?

What would this stance do for your enjoyment of the party?

In this metaphor, the party is life, and Norma represents your pain – all the unwelcome emotions / sensations / thoughts / memories / urges that show up as part of being alive and human. Would you be willing to welcome those into your life, even if you don't like them?

How is Norma like your pain?

Do you hide your pain away? Try to talk it away? Yell at it?

Would it help you to welcome, and to willingly accept, that pain if it meant you could live your life more fully, if you could "enjoy your party"?

What might happen if you got to know your pain more fully, just as you would if you got to know Norma?

I invite you to give it a go! Imagine one part of your pain is a person. What would they look like? How would they dress? What would their voice sound like? How might they smell? What kind of hairdo does your pain have?

Norma's story is helpful because it suggests to us the alternative of letting go, of being willing to be present with our experience as it is, rather than living our lives trying to escape our pain or giving up on ourselves.

Another word for willingness is acceptance. Watch out here! The kind of acceptance I'm talking about is NOT resignation. In *Get Out of Your Mind and into Your Life: the New Acceptance and Commitment Therapy* (2005), Steve Hayes talks about where the word "acceptance" originates: from the Latin "capere" which means "to take". Acceptance as it's meant in Acceptance and Commitment Therapy (ACT) is an active thing. Acceptance is where you might take a pen someone hands to you, rather than resigning and allowing the pen to be thrown at you, believing you have no other choice. Don't believe me? Try for yourself. Here are some comparisons that you might use to begin to get closer to accepting the parts of your experience and your pain which you cannot change:

Willingness is ...

- Like riding with your pain, the way you might take the training wheels off the bike and pedal away, knowing you need to risk falling in order to balance.
- Holding hands with your pain, the way a nurse holds the hand of a suffering patient.
- Allowing your pain to be as it is, as John Lennon sings in 'Let it Be'.
- Appreciating your pain, the way an artist eventually appreciates the paint that accidentally spilled over their best painting because it forced them to create something new and different.
- Exploring your pain, the way a baby explores a new toy.
- Getting to know your pain the way you would reconnect with a treasured old friend who you haven't seen for years.
- Cupping your pain gently in your hands, the way you'd hold a delicate precious plant you are repotting.
- Watching what happens with your pain in different situations, the way you might watch oil shimmer on the surface of water as the wind plays over it and raindrops fall upon the puddle.

- Walking with your pain the way a cyclist walks their bike when it has a puncture.
- Hearing your pain speak the way a truth and reconciliation tribunal would listen to the story of a long-oppressed sufferer of a brutal regime.

Acceptance versus resignation

It's important to discover that there are some subtle, but important, differences between letting go and resigning yourself to something (or giving up).

Let's think about this another way. To do this, you might need to fast forward to the future in your mind's eye. Imagine that you've just cleaned the house, you're wearing some nice new clothes and you're ready to go out through the door. Your child has been playing outside really happily, rolling around in a bit of mud – but that's okay because the babysitter is about to show up. But then, suddenly, the child falls over and hurts themselves. You hear the scream and then a moment later they come running in through the back door, desperately wanting you to give them a cuddle and make everything all right.

At that moment, would you yell, 'Get out of my house, you're covered in mud'? Or would you allow them to traipse that mud through the house so that they can get what they need in that moment: a great big hug?

Welcoming that dirty child into your arms is a great example of what we mean when we talk about willingness. It means being willing to have something as it is. That's not the same as wanting to have it. It's about not struggling or fighting, and just allowing it to be there when it is there.

As you've probably already noticed from reading Sonya's story, and as you've worked through your own experiences, it is often the case that the more we fight these difficult emotions and feelings, the more they pop out at times when we least expect or need them. This doesn't mean that by allowing yourself to feel these things, it's going to get rid of them in any way. But I'd encourage you to have a go at allowing them in and taking this new stance, so that you start thinking, *'Okay, there you are'* when they come back. Just allow yourself to feel curious about them.

Try it and see what kind of change this might bring to your life. This is an important part of letting go of the struggle and making space for those things that are so hard for us. When you get used to doing this, you will see that it is a really helpful step along the way to greater acceptance of the things you think and feel.

The difficult part about this is that you can't do it in half measures. It's a bit like being pregnant - you're either pregnant or you're not; you can't be half pregnant. When it comes to being willing, you're either willing or you're not.

If you're sneakily trying to be willing in order to get rid of something, are you really being willing? Are you really being open to that thing showing up in your life? Probably not.

You can make choices about how long you choose to be willing for. At any point, you're welcome to go back to what you did before. If you continually used to fight or struggle, you know that option is still there, we're not taking it away from you. And you also have the chance to discover that every moment of trying willingness opens up new opportunities and options for you.

SECTION 7

BECOME AWARE

Have you ever driven somewhere and realised you had no memory of how you got there? For most of us, this is a regular occurrence; we spend a lot of our days hardly noticing what is going on. But one of the benefits of bringing yourself more into the present moment is noticing what is actually happening right now. It gives us the opportunity to be more present in the moment. Often, what's happening right here, right now offers us more opportunities than we might have realised. That's because we are so used to living in the world of our thoughts.

If you thought mindfulness was just a kind of meditation technique where you have to slow down and pay attention to your breath – and that hasn't worked for you it might be worth you trying some of these other kinds of mindfulness that I'll share with you now.

MINDFULNESS OF EATING CHOCOLATE

Next time you're ready for a treat, grab your chocolate and give this exercise a go.

To begin, divide the piece of chocolate you're going to eat into two pieces. Then, eat the first half exactly as you would normally do it. Go ahead and do it now. Enjoy!

Now, hold the other piece of chocolate in your hand. As you're holding the chocolate, see if you can notice its texture under your fingers. Perhaps your fingers are cold, and you can feel the smoothness of the chocolate. Perhaps your hands are warm, and you can feel the chocolate beginning to melt underneath your fingers.

Go ahead, take the chocolate in your hand and see what you notice.

Next, bring the chocolate up to your nose and have a sniff. What does the chocolate smell like? Does it smell sweet? Creamy? Bitter? Perhaps it has a different kind of smell. You can inhale the aroma that comes from the chocolate and really notice it, even if you can't quite put words on the particular aromas you're picking up.

Now, notice how your body is starting to react to this chocolate. Have you begun to salivate? Are you fighting the urge to put it in your mouth?

If you can, hold off putting the chocolate in your mouth just yet! Stay with the urge and notice it. Keep exploring the texture and the aroma and the anticipation of eating the chocolate. Hold the chocolate up to the light and see what you notice. Does it reflect the light or absorb the light? Now that you're looking at it so closely, can you spot anything you've not noticed before about the surface of the chocolate? Are there indentations and shadows? See if you can look at this chocolate in the way that a curious scientist would look at chocolate, as though you were encountering it for the very first time.

Now, still noticing the urge to put the chocolate in your mouth, bring it closer to your ear. Moving it around in your fingers, see if the chocolate has a sound. Now, I know this might seem a bit random – and your mind might be busily telling you that this is a very strange thing to do! If it does, bring your focus straight back to the chocolate itself, and now, bring it to your lips. Try rubbing it against your lips. How does that feel compared with how it felt in your fingers? Does the chocolate melt onto your lips, or does it stay solid?

And now ... at the point of your own choosing – and not acting on the urge to eat the chocolate all at once – put the chocolate into your mouth and hold it there. Move it around a little in your mouth, but resist the urge to bite down on it. Notice how it feels in different parts of your mouth. Try it on your tongue and see if the taste of the chocolate changes. Notice how the chocolate feels against your teeth, and again, notice that urge to bite down. See if you can just hold off a bit longer while you notice that urge. And then, when you choose, you can bite down. Try to pay attention to what that feels like ...

Was there an explosion of flavour? Or was it just the same? Does the chocolate taste as sweet as you'd anticipated? Or did you notice any other flavours in it?

As you start to swallow, see if you can notice the beginning of the swallow, right down to the end when you can't feel the chocolate anymore. Carry on eating the chocolate slowly and really observantly. If you find your mind wandering, pull it gently back to the experience of eating this chocolate.

When you've finished chewing and swallowing, notice what taste lingers in your mouth. Run your tongue over your teeth – can you feel any tiny remnants of chocolate that are left?

As you observe these things notice also if you feel an urge to have more chocolate, or whether you actually feel quite sated after the chocolate you've had. Try not to judge, just notice what you're experiencing right now, and allow it to be as it is. Whenever you feel ready, you can stop this exercise and carry on with your day.

So what did you notice?

In your observations, did you contrast the experience of eating the chocolate on autopilot with eating it slowly and mindfully? If you didn't, try to have a bit of a think about that now. Which experience felt more fulfilling? Which experience did you discover more from? Which experience did you like better?

Don't feel as if you have to like the mindful part of the exercise better. There are some parts of it that are not that appealing. You might not like the texture of melted chocolate on your fingers. You might not particularly like feeling as if you're covered in melted chocolate. You might even prefer the quick satisfying crunch of chocolate as you eat it straightaway. And of course, that's all okay. You're allowed to have those preferences. The purpose of this exercise is not necessarily to enjoy the chocolate more - although sometimes that does happen - it's about noticing the experience.

Play around with it a little bit. If you're someone who enjoys eating chocolate quickly, see if you can eat quickly and mindfully.

You can try some more mindful eating exercises too. How about trying it with something you don't particularly enjoy? What happens when you slow that process right down? I've tried it with brussels sprouts! It can be really interesting - I discovered some things I didn't know about brussels sprouts before.

You can also do it with your tea or coffee. This is a good one as, for many of us, as it's something we do at several points through the day. So it can become a sort of mindfulness check-in for you. A moment to slow down and notice what is actually happening in the here and now - and just allowing it to be as it is.

MINDFULNESS OF FEEDING YOUR BABY

Let's relate mindfulness to your baby now. Our next exercise is mindfulness about feeding your baby, and it works for either breastfeeding or bottle-feeding. Set yourself up to feed your baby as you normally would, and as you settle into the feeding, just take a few moments to notice your breath. Think about where you feel your breath most strongly in this moment. Notice the sensations of your body resting on whatever surface it's resting on right now. Is it hard or soft? Cool or warm? Begin to drop into the moment.

Because this exercise involves interaction with another being – your baby – you need to bring a little bit of extra flexibility to it. At any point it's okay to stop what you're doing and attend to your baby's needs. With that in mind, begin to tune in to what's happening in the present moment, as you feed your baby. Start by noticing the places in your body that are in contact with your baby's body. Think about it as if you could draw a line around the places you're in contact with. This could be around your belly, or where your arm supports the baby's neck and head, or, if you're breastfeeding, it could be your breast in the baby's mouth. Perhaps your baby holds onto your finger or rests their arm on your chest.

Just see if you can experience this connection without needing to judge it. Note the temperature. Observe if you can notice any textures. Bring in your focus on any textures you can feel. Gently rub your fingers over the surface of your baby's outfit or across their skin. Feel the warm or cool sensations, the rough or smooth textures. If your mind begins to wander, just bring yourself gently back to the sensations you're feeling and the sounds you can hear as they feed – all the little snorting and sucking sounds. Notice what other noises are there. Perhaps there are some subtler, quieter noises you've not heard before. There may even be louder noises when your baby stops because they're windy. Whatever noise is there, try to hear it as if you're listening to a new piece of music, rather than just another noise.

Using your sense of sight, notice some things about your baby that you maybe haven't explored before. A good place to start is by looking at their ear. Explore the shape of your baby's ear. Notice where it's rounded, where it's thicker and thinner, maybe even where it's translucent. Focus on the play of light and shade around your baby's ear. Can you see tiny hairs growing on the surface of your baby's skin? Or is it entirely smooth? Zoom out a little and look at your baby's ear in the context of their whole head and make eye contact. Look into your baby's eyes as they meet yours and, as best you can, stay focused on the sensing, the seeing, and the noticing. Notice the patterns of your baby's hair, where it begins and ends, notice the curls and the straight parts, the colour and the texture.

Breathe in through your nose and see what you can smell right now. Perhaps you can smell that baby kind of smell – perhaps you can smell the milk. Or perhaps you can smell that your baby's nappy needs changing! Whatever's there, try to approach it without judgement. Notice the characteristics of that smell – is it sour or sweet, bitter or floral? Whatever kind of smell it is, just try to experience it without judging it.

Notice this connection you have with your baby as they feed. Sit for a few moments and see if you can truly experience the sights, the smells, and the sounds and sensations that are around you right now.

Notice what's happening inside of you ... What emotions are you experiencing as you sit with your baby? There could be a variety of emotions emerging. It may even be scary for you to experience what it's like to be with your baby. You may feel a sense of connection and love, or you might feel exhaustion. Whatever emotion is there, try to practise just being with it, and noticing at the same time the sensation of holding your baby in this way.

Think about what your thoughts are doing. You've probably had thousands of thoughts since we started. Whatever your thoughts are, keep bringing your mind back to the present, noticing what's actually happening, rather than what your mind tells you is happening. If your mind wanders a thousand times, bring it back a thousand times. Don't worry, you're not doing it wrong, this is the process of mindfulness. This is how it works – it is the process of learning to bring your attention back to something.

Bring your attention back to your baby, and to all those sensations that you notice – the feeling of the baby in your arms, the sounds you're hearing – while still doing whatever your baby needs in that moment. And then, when you and your baby are ready, you can finish the exercise and carry on with your day.

What did you notice with this exercise?

How might you start to bring mindfulness into your day-to-day life? When will you practise again?

MINDFULNESS OF WATCHING YOUR BABY

Here's another mindfulness exercise to do with your baby. As they get bigger, you can do this when they begin to move around and play a bit more. Begin by settling your baby when they're in one of their waking phases in a space where they can play safely with minimal intervention from you. (It's absolutely fine at any point to respond to your baby if they need you. Be guided by them.)

The rest of the time, take a space and sit alongside your baby on the floor. Begin with a couple of deep breaths. See if you can notice where the breath enters your body and where it leaves your body. Perhaps it's at your mouth or at your nose. Perhaps you feel it going deep down into your chest and past there into your stomach. Or maybe it's higher up, at the top of your diaphragm. Either way is fine. Just notice where your breath is right now.

Expand out from where you feel your breath most strongly to observe the outside world, looking around the room, and seeing your baby there next to you. See if you can sense both your breath and the feeling of the floor underneath you. Notice where your baby is – are they close to you, or further away? What is that like for you? What emotions are you experiencing right now? What sensations can you feel?

Watch your baby as they begin to play or move in some way. Notice how their body moves and how they interact with objects around them. Is there anything new or different that you haven't observed about these interactions before? See if you can wait patiently without having to do anything for your infant unless they need you to. See if you can observe the way they explore the objects around them and the world around them. Do they use their hands, their mouth, their feet, or another part of their body? Do they roll, curl, crawl, or toddle?

How calm is your child right now? Are they very involved in what they're doing? Or is your baby all over the place – moving from one thing to the other? Again, if you notice judgements emerging, just observe those thoughts. Bring yourself back to where you are right now, watching your baby. It's perfectly natural for your focus to wander. That's okay. Just keep bringing yourself back to this visual contact with your baby in the room.

As you continue to watch your baby, perhaps you'll notice that they do a kind of circling motion. They might go out and explore for a while and then come back and seek you out. Or maybe not. Just observe what they do and how your baby responds to you sitting here patiently watching them. You'll probably find that along the way, you'll have an urge to say something to your baby. To delight in something with them. To comment on what they're doing. Maybe even to give them a warning that perhaps you're aware they've heard before and know about already.

If it's not endangering the safety of your baby, give it a go and see if you can hold back on giving them that warning. See if you can notice the words as they form in your mind and the urge that you've got to say it. It might be an urge that's very pleasant – you might be very excited and driven to enjoy with them whatever they're working on. You might feel a strong level of concern. As long as your baby is safe, see if you can hold that urge. Notice what happens when you don't interrupt, or when you don't let yourself enjoy what they're doing along with them.

This isn't about how you should or shouldn't be parenting. And in no way is this mindfulness exercise instructing you to do this all of the time. This is about taking a break from the constant cycle of things you have to do as a mother and focusing a little on the importance of simply *being* as a mother – having that opportunity to just notice before you choose what you do.

Coming back to the urge to respond to your baby in some way, allow yourself to make a choice once you've sat with the urge for a little while. You can choose whether you want to continue in this observer stance, watching your baby, or whether you'd like to enter into that moment with them. Maybe you want to move closer to them, make eye contact with them and join in as they explore their new toy or their new situation. Or maybe you choose to stay sitting back and continue watching. You can keep doing this for quite a few minutes: stopping, waiting, watching, and observing what's happening for you.

Check in at regular intervals to bring your attention onto what your baby is doing and what's happening inside of you. At these times, see if you can be present with allowing whatever desires emerge. See if you can stay present with that, without having to change, alter, fix or avoid them.

It's also okay to just do this for little moments at any point during the day. It doesn't have to be a long exercise. Just see what you learn by pulling back and watching and observing this baby that you have in your life right now.

FLEXIBLY DROPPING INTO MINDFULNESS

Most of the exercises that I've introduced to you in this chapter have been fairly long and involved and that's not necessarily how mindfulness has to be. One of the useful skills that you can learn from a more formal mindfulness practice is this skill of dropping into the moment.

I imagine this as being a little bit like a parachutist dropping in to support you. And it's like a reminder to you to drop into the present to take a moment to just stop and observe. Give yourself space to notice whatever's happening. We spend so much of our life on autopilot or just responding, based on the stress we might feel. Often, we don't stop to notice what's really happening for us in any given moment. Often, we don't stop to observe sights, sounds, smells, tastes, and textures.

Sometimes we just need to check in with ourselves and observe how we're doing.

This can become a precious and helpful thing to do. It's only when you drop into the moment that you can choose to do what you wish to do in that moment. You see that you have the opportunity to connect with what matters to you in the long term rather than just doing things because they seem to be the obvious things to do, or because it's what you've always done.

So, I suggest you think about applying mindfulness to some frequent activities that you do, or places you visit during the day. Some examples could be brushing your teeth, making a meal, doing the washing up, or putting dishes away. How about the mindfulness of changing nappies? That can be a mind-broadening experience!

The more you do this, the more skilful you'll get at becoming aware of yourself. You may also discover new and interesting things that you might not have known about your environment. Along with this, recognising what you're grateful for at a given time or day is a very well-established technique for helping to improve mood and helping you to live more effectively with your anxiety. It can help you feel more connected to the people around you.

Go on, give it a try. You'll learn mindfulness best by just doing it.

You'll find a list overleaf of all the different options you have for how you might practise and learn some mindfulness along the way. Have a look through the list and circle the ones that appeal to you. Then choose one that you can make a start on right now. See if you can carve out ten minutes today to do this. Keep doing it for long enough – maybe even a couple of weeks – until you've had a chance to see if it works for you.

Always remember that the purpose of mindfulness is not to get rid of things or to be calmer, it's about being in the present and noticing things that are already here.

- Mindfulness of watching my baby
- Mindfulness of breathing
- Five senses mindfulness
- Downloading an app to learn mindfulness
- Getting a book or CD out of the library
- Downloading mp3 tracks to guide your mindfulness
- Doing three-minute check-ins
- Attaching mindfulness to changing nappies
- Attaching mindfulness to a regular thing you do every day
- Taking a specific time during the day when you try to notice what's happening

So, which of these things will you commit to doing? When will you start? What might the barriers be – and how might you work with and around these barriers?

What will you do if you find that you haven't done this?

Give it a go ...

TWO SHINY BOTTLES

Let's practise some choosing now. I'm going to offer you two shiny bottles of magical potions. You've got to make a choice which one you take – one or the other ...

One bottle gives you total control over how your child turns out. It allows you to entirely determine what their future will be like – their career, their health, their prosperity, their success. The only catch? If you choose the potion in this bottle, you don't get to be there. You jump miraculously to your child in their mid-twenties.

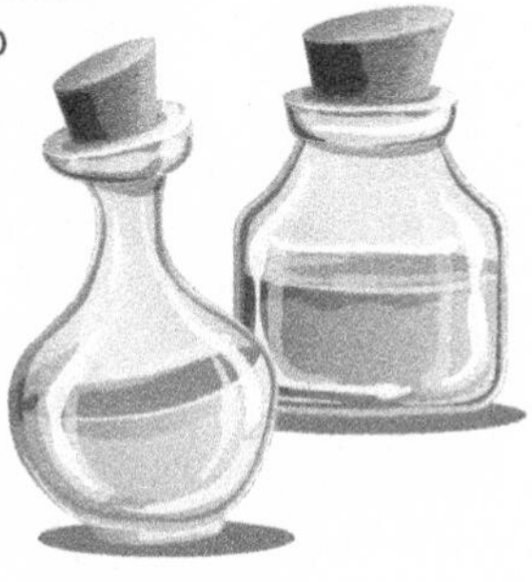

The second bottle is just as shiny and interesting. This bottle allows you to choose to experience absolutely everything that happens with your children with no control whatsoever over the outcome.

If you choose the second bottle, you get to experience all the highs and lows, the joys and the sorrows, the love and the hatred – and all the other incredible things that might happen as your child develops.

Which bottle would you choose?

I'm sorry. Of course, there is no potion that will ensure your child's future success and prosperity. (Although I'm sure there would have been a number of parents over the years that would have been prepared to take it!)

This metaphor is helpful in that it illustrates the difference between process versus outcome. Often in our lives we are so quick and willing to sacrifice everything for control over the outcome, rather than allowing ourselves the flexibility to enjoy the journey. That's a shame, because sometimes the journey can be the richest part.

What would it mean for you if you were to choose that second bottle?

How would it change the things you do day-to-day?

Would it allow you a few moments to leave the dishes in the sink, make an easy dinner and enjoy some time with your child?

If you struggled when it came to choosing your values, remember that using mindfulness and thinking about the journey, rather than the destination, can be a helpful way of moving you forward in being able to choose the values that matter to you.

SECTION 8

BECOMING A SOUP MUM AND MAKING SPACE FOR YOURSELF WITH YOUR THOUGHTS

One of the problems of being human and having a mind is that we get caught up in our thoughts and see things through the prism of our thoughts. Perhaps you're aware of this happening to you, or perhaps not. Let me give you an example. If you have the thought, *I'm a bad mother*, and then try to counter that with the fifteen things you've done today that make you a good mother, then before you know it, you're in a fight with your thoughts. As soon as that happens, you can find yourself constantly preoccupied with your thoughts, which takes you out of your life and out of your in-the-moment experience with your baby. There's a gesture for this: if you hold one hand in a fist and the other hand smacks over the top of the fist, fusing with it, it shows you what we're like when we're fused with our thoughts (this is called cognitive fusion).

This chapter is about ways you can help yourself to become defused from your thoughts (cognitive defusion). You will discover how to give yourself time to *choose* how you act, rather than having to act in a way that's dictated by your thoughts or your feelings – or having to escape the thoughts, feelings, or sensations inside you that cause you such pain.

Here in New Zealand, we have a synonym for getting drunk ... we call it "getting trollied"! The bonus is that it doesn't even involve a swear word. But you can apply the word to something else. I have a story about this that may seem familiar to you ...

I'm at the supermarket with my list in hand, putting groceries in my trolley as I move around the aisles. But as I go, I notice several items calling out to me from the shelves. There are some chips (crisps) on special offer, and a delicious new chocolate bar. There are some succulent-looking grapes that are certainly healthier, but still not on my list. Before I know it, all these things and more end up in my trolley. And they stay in my trolley, even though I know there's a very good chance that I might bump into someone I know. If that happens, I know I'll probably experience some supermarket-related shame due to the fact that I've got a trolley laden with chips, treats, and chocolate.

I get to the checkout and load the treats onto the conveyer belt. They go through the till and I load them into my bags, put them in the trolley, carry them out to my car, then into my pantry, and sooner or later, put them into my stomach.

Isn't this fascinating? At any point along the way, there were plenty of opportunities for me not to keep those chips and chocolates. I could have stopped at the point where they started calling to me from the shelf. I could have stopped at the point I put them in my trolley. I could have stopped at the point they were in the trolley and put them back on the shelf. I could have stopped at the point of putting them on the conveyer belt and said, 'No thank you!' I could even have stopped after I'd bought them and taken them to the customer services desk and returned them for a refund. I could have stopped and left them in my pantry and decided not to eat them. And yet, I didn't. I didn't do any of these things.

Part of this is because once we start doing something, we don't tend to think about it very hard. The thinking process is like that. Once we start thinking, we don't think very hard about the impact those thoughts have upon us. We tend to take them as truths and just act accordingly.

You can do the same things that I do with chips and chocolate with your thoughts. When they show up, they might pull you in. They might talk to you in some way, like the chocolate did with me. You might put them in your trolley. You might believe and act on your thought without even noticing it, without even realising that you had a choice not to.

You can go around acting as if the thought that you are a bad mother is actually a fact, like a tangible reality that you can actually touch. Have you ever been able to touch that thought?

Before you know it, you've bought the thought hook, line and sinker. It's there with you very frequently. And it's a bit like there's a special offer on it: *Check it out! Bad mother – two for the price of one today!*

But here's the cool part – even though you might have got trollied on the thought initially, you can still return to the thought and see if it's actually helpful to have it in your trolley.

Next time you go to that metaphorical supermarket and find yourself getting pulled by a thought, you can notice what's happening – notice the pull of that thought and leave it on the shelf. You didn't get trollied!

You can notice when you're carrying the thought around and acting based on that thought – you still didn't get trollied. You noticed.

You can even return it after the fact and say, 'Hang on, thank you, I don't actually need that thought. It's not really helping me very much.' Your mind might be a little surprised, but it's worth a try. This isn't about arguing with the thought, or getting rid of it, it's just about noticing when it shows up and not getting trollied all the time!

Let's try an exercise. Take a moment to consider what you know about saliva and why it's useful ...

Perhaps you were aware that museums use chemically identical saliva to clean their exhibits because it's such an effective cleaning agent. Or maybe you knew that saliva helps to protect our teeth and pre-digest our food. Saliva is pretty useful stuff!

Now I'd like you to do something that might seem totally unrelated. Take a moment and picture the most beautiful wine glass or goblet that you can imagine. Now bring your attention and your focus to the saliva that's in your mouth. Just notice it there. Imagine collecting this saliva and spitting it into the glass. And then, collect more saliva and spit that into the glass, and go on repeating this until you have a wine glass full of your saliva. And now ... I'd like you to imagine drinking it.

How do you feel right now?

Every time I do this exercise, I feel an incredibly strong sense of disgust, and feel sick to my stomach. And there's a good chance you'll feel the same. But this is an interesting reaction.

Think about it – did you actually drink the saliva? Was the goblet actually there? No. The power of your thoughts can make you experience this strength of feeling. Now that I've helped you fuse with the idea of saliva as disgusting, let me help you defuse from it.

Ideally, do this exercise in a place where you don't mind speaking out loud for thirty seconds and don't mind sounding like an idiot! It is really worth a try.

So now I'd like you to say the word "saliva" over and over again, quite quickly, out loud, for thirty seconds. Get a timer and when you're ready, say it and keep saying it for the full thirty seconds.

Now, take a moment to notice what happened when you did the exercise. For example:

- What happened to the sound of the words?
- Where did your attention go?
- How much did you still perceive the meaning of the word as you were saying it?

This exercise can help us to get a little bit of space from the fused thought, to unhook a little bit from the thought. Now, let's try it again with something that's a little bit more loaded for you. Let's try it with the word "mother".

Begin by noticing what shows up when you think of the word "mother". Notice the feelings that are there. Notice the thoughts that are there. Observe the sensations in your body and then, when you're fully connected – possibly with quite a bit of pain that's associated with the word – see if you can do the same thirty-second exercise out loud, over and over again, and observe what happens.

What did you discover this time? Did you notice that you were able to get a little bit more space from the word? If you did, great. What would you like to do with that space?

If you didn't, that's okay. I'd encourage you to keep reading. Often, some of the exercises that work for some thoughts don't work so well for others, and vice versa. It's worth giving all the exercises a go and finding out which ones are best for the thoughts you're struggling with at this point.

Now, are you ready for something else quite random? Find a chair somewhere in your surroundings and look really carefully at it. Start by observing all the things you can notice about the chair:

- What colour is it?
- What shape is it?
- What kind of backrest does it have?
- Does it look comfortable to sit in?

Write down all of your thoughts, feelings and associations about the chair here.

Okay, so now you've created a network of what comes up for you when you think about the word "chair". It might contain judgements and evaluations, but it might also have quite a lot of description in it.

If you're willing, let's try another little experiment. Imagine that chair IS your pain. It's the low mood you feel, the anxiety you wake with during the night, the thoughts of how hard it is to cope, the feeling of butterflies in your stomach ... all the things that are hurting you right now. Imagine these woven into the fabric of that chair. What do you have to add into your network of associations now?

So, congratulations. Mazeltov! You've just experienced a very human experience: isn't it incredible that you can relate something as boring as a chair to all that stuff you've been struggling with? I'm betting you've never thought of a chair that way before in your life! Okay, so it probably feels more freaky than incredible. You know what? Your mind has already been busy doing this for you, all the time. It's the speciality of the mind. And once your mind associates something neutral with something painful, you're very likely to feel the pull of avoidance tugging at you.

Did you just shut your eyes? Turn away from the chair? Let's work with this a little bit and try something new. Rather than moving away from this chair, let's see if we can extend your network more. Practise allowing your feelings to be AS you are present with them AND noticing what's happening in the world, rather than being stuck inside your mind.

Now, stand up and literally turn the chair upside down. Observe what else you notice. Does it have anything written underneath it? Can you tell me the temperature of the different parts of the chair?

Okay, so now you've created a network of what comes up for you when you think about the word "chair."[2] It might contain judgements and evaluations, but it might also have quite a lot of description in it.

Let's move on to something a little bit more challenging. Let's come back to the word "mother" and look at this idea again. To begin with, think about all the things you noticed earlier on when the word came up. Jot them down – and as you do, you may notice some of the pain that you feel.

2 This ability humans have to relate one thing to another thing backwards and forwards really is actually amazing and incredible; no other animal can do it, and babies begin to be able to do it as they learn language. In fact, there's good evidence it's at the basis of how we learn language itself. The theory behind this is called Relational Frame Theory (Hayes, Barne-Holmes and Roacje (2001); Villatte, Villatte, and Hayes (2016)), and it's the theory that underpins Acceptance and Commitment Therapy. The awesome part is there is a lot of basic psychological science underpinning ACT, which gives us good evidence about how the processes you're learning in this book will help you.

It's really worth keeping going with this exercise. Just sit with it for a little bit and see if further things come up. See if you can make some associations that seem really random. You might come up with some associations connected with animals and their mothers, for example. Or even some more "sideways" associations, like milk, and the temperature of milk, and the smell of milk.

Imagine that you're a TV-show host, interviewing people on the street about the word "mother" ... what might they say? Keep at it, and try to go as wide and as broad as you possibly can. Notice what happens as you build these further associations. See if you can link off one of the words that you've already got there.

Here's an example of what happens for me when I think about the word "mother", and then, what I managed to come up with when I pushed my thinking sideways, upside down, and all around (the way that a small child might play with a toy – there was no putting it in my mouth, though!)

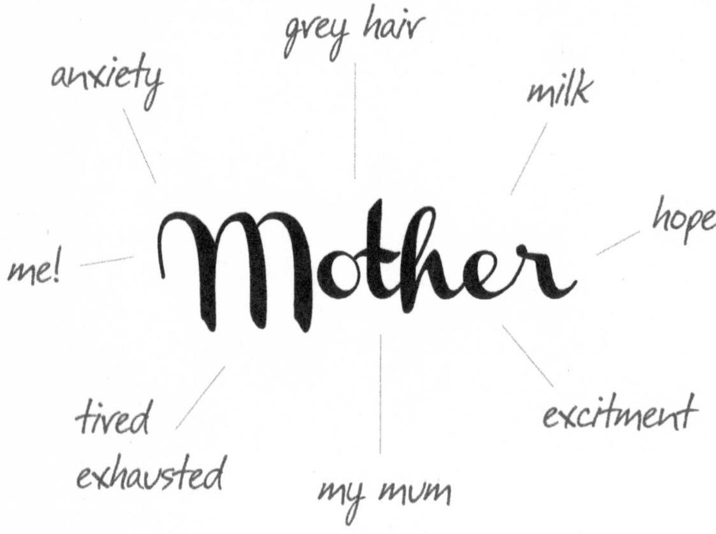

Figure 8: *My "mother" associations.*

See if you can find out for yourself whether this exercise allowed you to get a little bit unhooked from your fused thinking. Did it let you notice more? One of the interesting things about our thoughts is that once you've had a thought, you can't actually remove it. It's there. But don't just take my word for it. Check in with your own experience and see if it's true. A good example is when you learn a new word, or buy a new brand of car that you weren't aware of before. Suddenly, you start to see that car, or hear that word almost all over the place, even though you didn't know it existed previously. Isn't it amazing?

Afterwards, do you think you could forget that car or that word existed? Give it a go. See if you can forget a word that you've

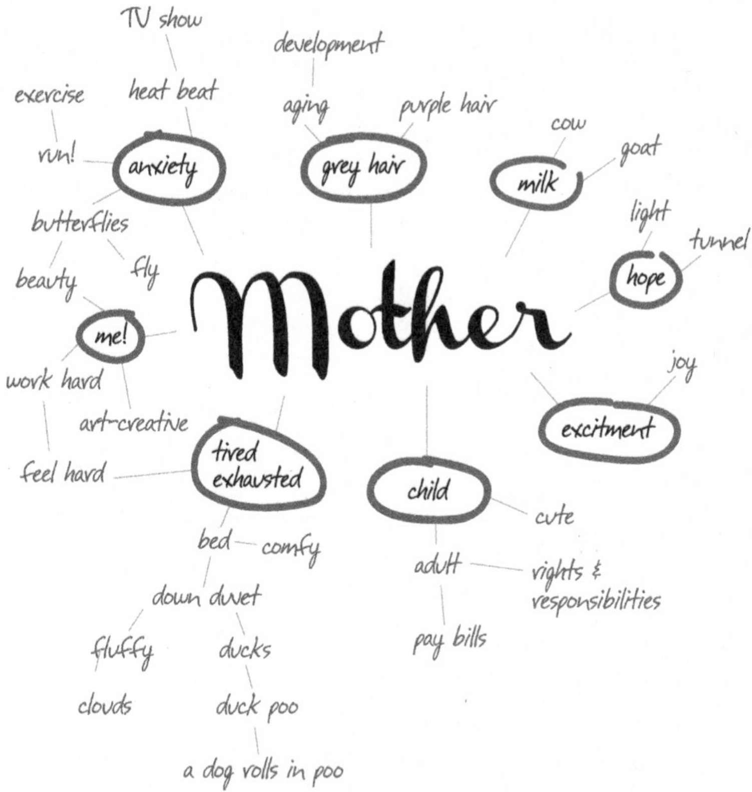

Figure 9: *My expanded, whacky, creative associations to 'mother'.*

recently learnt, or a brand of car, or an appliance you've just discovered. I'm guessing you'll find it really hard to do. That's because this is an important part of how our brains work. It's how we're so amazingly efficient at learning new information and learning really amazing things about how to keep ourselves safe, warm, dry, and fed.

So, let's pause for a moment and think about what this means for you ...

How often have you tried to get rid of a feeling or a word that shows up in your mind by trying to argue it away, or trying to forget that it's there by stuffing it down in the furthest reaches of your mind? If it's true that we can't get rid of things so easily – and there's some pretty good science to suggest that – then going further out and bringing in new associations is a pretty cool way of giving us the opportunity to choose, rather than be driven by this process that we call cognitive fusion.

So that's fusion. Let's try an exercise in defusion now. A good place to start is with lullabies. This is another verbal exercise, so you might want to be alone with your baby. Perhaps you've got a favourite lullaby that you like to sing to your baby that you associate with feeling nice and calm. Or maybe there's a lullaby that you remember from your own childhood. Now see if you can identify a thought that's been bothering you, one that you've fused with. This will be one of those thoughts that are hard to see beyond at times. Have a go at singing that thought to the tune of your favourite lullaby. You might feel like a bit of an idiot! But I'd recommend doing it in front of your baby, as it can be kind of funny. You'll know if it's working if it feels a little bit amusing. If you can't make it work with a lullaby, try it with one of your favourite pop songs, preferably something upbeat.

What did you discover? Now, this might be one of those exercises that you might be reluctant to do, but I'd really encourage you to give it a go. You might need to try it a few times, and then, hopefully, you'll see for yourself how effective it can be.

As you did before, notice what happens to the meaning of the words and the impact they had upon you when you sang the song. Were you able to get a bit of space from them to see them as just words, rather than commands that you're forced to do?

Next, we're going to move on to some more visual defusion strategies. This can be really useful if you have thoughts that show up as images in your mind rather than words. Imagine that you've got PowerPoint or a slides program up on your computer. Visualise typing the thought that you're working on at the moment. Make it in a font that fits with the way you think about it. So you might want to make it big and bold or dripping red, and add an image or texture into the background that fits. There's an example for you below.

Now, bring up another slide and put the same words in. This time, put them in a colour that's exactly opposite the colour you feel for that thought. So for example, if it's a very dark or blue

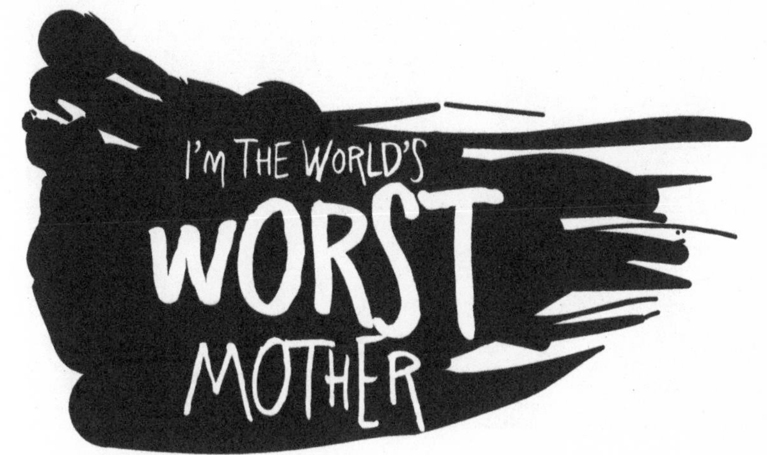

I'm the worlds
Worst Mother

thought, you might choose to put them in a bright orange or yellow. Then put them in a font that really doesn't fit the way you feel about that thought. Then, add in some images. Maybe you can "go broad" like you did earlier. Maybe you've got some images or ideas that show up around this thought. You could maybe even animate the words so that they move around in a strange way. Notice how you feel when you look at the first slide and what happens when you look at the second. See if you can allow that image of the second slide to come up alongside the first slide when that difficult thought comes up.

You can do this using real materials as well, for example a collage.

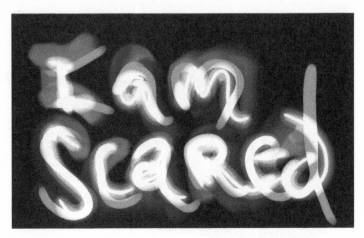

Figure 10a: *Kathryn's visual example of fusion with 'scared.'*

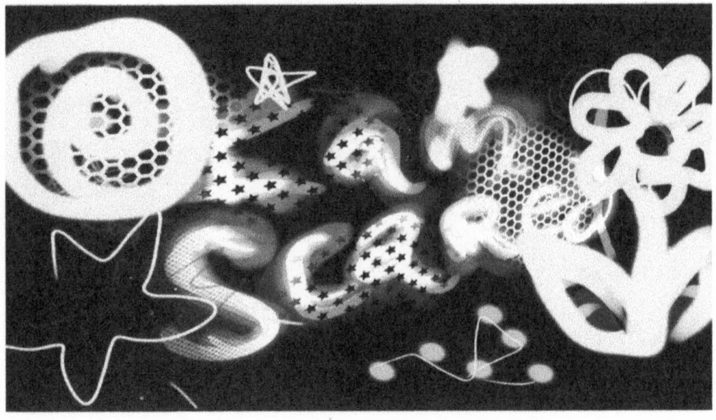

Figure 10b: *Kathryn's visual example of defusion from 'scared' by adding in new and incongruous images.*

If the thought is an image, there's another thing you can do. There are lots of apps that allow you to put pictures on top of photos. So if you can photograph the image that disturbs you, or if you can find a picture or a piece of art that fits, then try using the app to put a picture on top of that image. For example, if I was bothered by thoughts that I might harm my dog, I might take a picture of my dog and then add funny ears onto my dog. Or I might put a shark fin on him, or put stars bursting out of his tail. And then when I have that thought show up about wanting to harm my dog, I can remember that image, or take another look at it to give me a little bit of space so that I don't see that thought of harming my dog as a command or a prediction. It will help me take a step back and recognise it as just a thought, like any other random thought I have. It's only as serious as a thought about stars coming out of my dog's tail.

There are tons and tons of defusion strategies. You might have success with some of your own. And I'd also suggest that there are ones that you can use quietly, in the privacy of your own mind if you happen to be out shopping, or on the bus. For example, you can imagine your thoughts coming out of the mouth of a political figure that you can't possibly take seriously. Or you could imagine your thoughts on the front page of a less reputable newspaper or magazine that you'd approach with scepticism. See if you can get yourself to the point where you find it really amusing, or you can feel a large sense of distance from those thoughts.

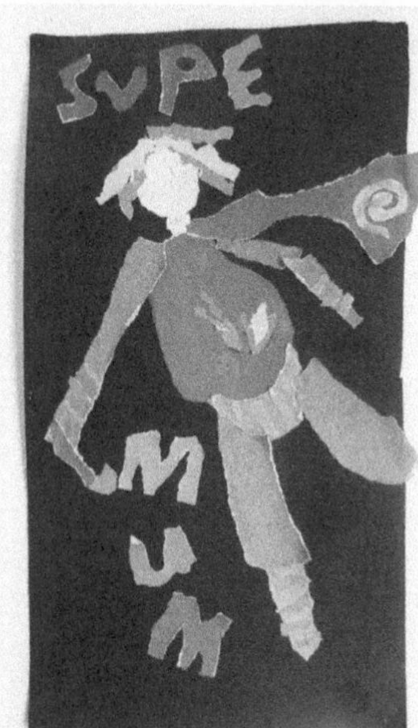

SUPE MUM

Many mothers get caught up in how others evaluate them. They sense they need to be a kind of "Super Mum". Sonya and I worked with this in her therapy. We devised a cool image to help her disentangle from the need to act perfectly in order to maintain a mask and the respect of others. This was especially important when doing that was at such great cost to herself. We imagined that maybe Super Mum had lost an "r" and become Supe Mum, AKA Soup Mum.

Supe Mum is the kind of mother who has a pot of soup on the boil on the stove, adding a few vegetables every day to extend the soup further. She wears unmatched socks and clothes, and her tummy bulges out like many women who have had a baby. Supe Mum uses the time she saves on being perfect and cooking perfect meals to do what she needs to do for herself – and takes the time to be with her kids. This is one example of defusion on a larger scale: it's defusion from one of the ways we think about a larger part of ourselves, rather than just defusion from a thought we might have.

Let's recap. Defusion is about allowing us enough space from our thoughts to make choices that allow us to act in the way that we want to act. As you'll have noticed from Sonya's story, it takes practise to get good at it. And you'll find that different strategies work for different kinds of thoughts.

Defusion can also open up ways for us to become more willing and less fixated on getting rid of the things that make our life difficult. It gives us the space we need to make room for these thoughts to show up, while also embracing the experiences that can allow us to grow.

SECTION 9

THE EVEN BIGGER PICTURE: FINDING A SPACE FROM WHICH TO ACT

Imagine yourself on a dark night, lying on some soft ground and looking up at the night sky. It's so clear and you can see multitudes of stars. You hear the sounds of the night around you, and you begin to notice that some stars are harder to see than others. It can take a little while for your eyes to adjust. Imagine as you look up that each star is like a kind of you: the mother you, the sister you, and you as a worker / teacher / learner / friend – each one twinkling brightly.

Sometimes it's like we get our telescope out and get stuck. It's true – there's an awful lot to see on one star alone, but as we fixate on one star out of billions, we lose sight of the larger, cosmic-sized reality here. There is so much more to us than just this one kind of self. So, let's zoom out again. Notice how the sky stretches out in all directions ... take in the infinity of space ... There's a part of you that's infinite like that.

Don't just believe me at face value; see if you can connect with this idea at the level of experience. If you're lucky, you'll have glimpsed this infinity of you before, stretching across space and time. If not, you can start to connect with it now. Observe how, at times, when the night is cloudy or when our surroundings demand our attention, how easily we lose sight of the many ideas of ourselves. Observe how we become hooked up by one kind of idea about ourselves. We fight against our own experiences and our feelings – it's a bit like a galactic struggle between planets orbiting our stars. We lose sight of the bigger picture. When we get caught up with the roles we play in life, we forget it is possible to look at these roles and *at* our struggles, rather than just looking out *from* them. It's as if we're standing on that planet that's about to be bombarded by a meteorite within that solar system that we're so caught up in.

Now, gently bring yourself back to lying there on the soft ground, staring up at the whole night sky. Notice, from your own experience, that there's far more to you than just the few stars in the constellation that you've previously described as yourself.

See if you can allow this experience to help you let go a little further, so that you're less caught up in the way you think about and define yourself, and then how you act upon it. Try to be safe in the knowledge that there is far more to you than you realised before.

I now invite you to think about – and do some work around – different kinds of self that you know about. You might even discover some new parts of yourself that you weren't aware of before. Firstly, begin by identifying the different stars in your night sky – the different roles that you take on in life. See if you can identify any of the ones that were mentioned in that exercise, or perhaps there are others. If you need some help, here are some examples:

Self as:

worker

mother

sister

friend

artist

adventurer

dreamer

shy person

fast thinker

WHAT FITS TOGETHER?

There are constellations of stars, and often there are constellations of different kinds of selves that make sense and seem to fit together, e.g. our role as mother, daughter, sister often go together in a family constellation. You might notice that there are some parts of yourself that don't necessarily fit into any constellation. Take a moment to notice – are these parts of you that you struggle or fight with? Are there parts of you that you would like to do more with, or to expand more? Maybe you can even find a new constellation that they will fit into that you didn't even know was there.

Why not jot down these kinds of self here:

THINK BACK ACROSS TIME

What stars have been there in the past? What roles or versions of yourself have you played that you don't play any longer?

Jot them down here ...

WHAT HELPS YOU?

Zoom out. What helps you look at the whole sky? What helps you see everything you are, beyond all these different kinds of self; beyond the everyday struggles?

Try to think about what activities you do that help you – they can be quite hard to identify at first, but stick with it. Any ideas you can come up with will be incredibly useful.

For example, I always feel much more in tune with where I am in the world when I'm on my mountain bike. It forces me to keep my attention on both my balance and the route that I'm taking – always being aware of where I am. This helps me to be fully present in the moment, and to really notice all the parts of me, while also being me.

Other people find this experience in religion or in an activity that gives them a sense of flow, maybe something creative. Other times, people can notice it just by stopping and noticing the difference between themselves and the things they're looking at.

Write your ideas down about the things that help you here:

STEPPING BACK

Notice the sky, and the space of the universe in this metaphor: while it holds and contains all the stars, it doesn't influence what happens to the stars and what happens between them. In a similar kind of way, this part of yourself – this observer self – doesn't have to have the same investment or influence in your struggles and emotions as the part of you that contains and holds these things. It is connected to them, but doesn't necessarily have to be controlling them. Just as the stars move around in their own way across the aeons of time, so this part of yourself can help you to notice, observe, and be present with the experiences you have, without the need to have to get involved in that struggle.

PUTTING EXPANSIVENESS INTO ACTION

Now, let's connect all this with some of the things you're struggling with right now. Where in your life do you think it could help you to practise this bigger thinking, this sense of expansiveness? How can the observer part of you help?

See if you can link this with the values and the things you care about. Maybe there's something you've been trying to do that you've been struggling with. Perhaps it's been about getting out and doing something when you've felt low. You might have felt like you wanted to give something a try to see if it might make a positive difference to your mood in service of your health and sustainability. Perhaps there's a phone call that you need to make that you've been dreading. Maybe it's writing a text message to connect with a friend, in service of going towards your values of friendship.

Whatever it is that might bring out that struggle, write it down and write down the activity you'd like to do to go along with it.

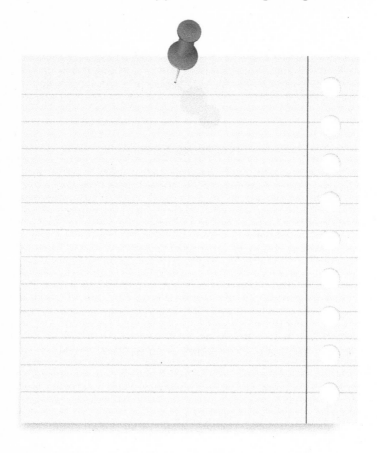

How confident are you that you'll be able to do this thing? On a scale where 0 = "completely unconfident and there's no way I'll do it", and 10 = "absolutely confident, I'm going off to do it right now", rate your own level of confidence here:

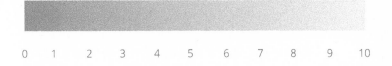

Figure 11: *Level of confidence scale.*

See if you can get yourself to seven out of ten on the confidence scale that you're going to be able to do this thing. And if it feels too big, scale it back a bit. Make it easier, maybe just start by finding the number for the phone call, or going outside your front door for thirty seconds.

Once you've written it down, see if you can bring yourself back to that zoomed-out position of looking at these parts of you that you get hooked up with. One of the key ones here might be the perception of yourself as a really depressed mother. When you're in that space, it's probably very hard for you to consider doing things that don't fit into that constellation of things that characterise you as a depressed mother.

So, pause, zoom out and remember that there are all these parts of you. Just like the stars in the sky. There are many, many different roles that you've played in life, many roles you still have to play.

See if you can use the observer perspective to just take a step towards something you really care about, right now. Give it a go, then come back when you've had a try.

What happened when you acted from the observer perspective?

How did it go? What was it like?

Were you able to get into that observer space? Or was it hard for you to step back?

If it was too hard, go back and have another try. Just make it a bit easier for yourself this time. Bring into play the other skills you've learnt from this book. Be mindfully aware, use defusion to unhook from thought barriers, practise some acceptance of where you are right now – being kind to yourself about the need for change.

If you were able to give it a go, how was that? Did it work for you? Is this something you'd be willing to try again?

Go on – it's worth it.

ALL THESE DIFFERENT PARTS OF ME

Now that you've heard about the metaphor of the stars as different parts of yourself, here's an exercise that will help you take it a little bit further. It will help you create something to help you visualise how you can use the part of yourself that encompasses all your other aspects. It will help you let go a little bit more and take small steps towards what you really care about.

Begin by collecting together lots of little bits that will fit in a plastic bottle with a tight-fitting lid. For example, it could be small coins, little twigs or marbles – any little things that you might find around your home or garden. It needs to be something that will last in water. Pull together as many of these objects as you can. If you've got a black surface you can work on, that's even better.

Try scattering some of the little objects around a bit like stars in the night sky, and then think of some of the things you've been struggling with. You can use some of the things you've identified from earlier in the book, or you could just notice, right now, some of the little things that are hard for you.

Begin by allocating some of these painful things to the objects that you have put out in front of you. Try to place them, spatially, where they would be in relation to each other. So for example, say I'm noticing a really heavy feeling of sadness right now. I might assign a dirty coin to it, or a piece of dark Lego and pop that into position. Then I might notice that there's also a sense of guilt, and that connects in a way to some of my memories of things that have happened in the past. So I might place a piece of dark-coloured ribbon or a seed there to convey the idea of old things growing into new things. Or I might use a crumpled-up piece of wrapping paper for that sensation of being used in some way. All of these little things build up like stars in a constellation. They connect with one another.

Then I'm going to ask you focus on the feeling of not wanting something. Recognise what you normally do when these feelings show up. But rather than acting on the feeling, see if you can sit for long enough to observe what it is that you want to do. For example, say I had that memory about the bad times when I wasn't able to be the kind of parent I wanted to be. In that scenario, I might have an urge to talk back to myself and reassure myself that I've been a good parent in other ways. I might say to myself, 'But hang on, you've done this, this and this ... they were all really good things.' So I might assign an object to that talking-back-to-myself strategy. Perhaps a balloon, because it can grow bigger.

If I discover that I usually tidy up to try to make my environment look better around me, I'll find an object like a shiny coin to represent that and place it next to the balloon. Maybe sometimes I tell myself to just "buck up" and sparkle, or I talk to a friend who just tells me to get on with it. In that scenario, I might put some glitter there next to my balloon and my shiny coin. Notice how these things cluster into two groups. It's almost like you're going to fight one thing with the other.

Keep noticing the things that show up under the heading of things that are painful. And keep noticing the things that you do to try to get rid of the things that hurt, or make them better. You might also include some of the stars that you identified in the previous exercise, representing the parts of you that you use to fight this. For example, if I think of myself as a psychologist, I can easily put that with the "brighten up and get better" shiny coin – and then try to fight the part of myself that feels sad.

Perhaps I might have a concept of myself as a mother who isn't good enough. And that can go in the part with everything else that's sad. It's starting to feel like we've got a bit of an intergalactic war going on here between these two piles of things!

As you're doing this, begin to connect with what part of this scenario is you. Are you one of these experiences? Are you your feelings of sadness? What if you're not just those things? What if there's more to you than that? What else could you be in this scenario? Are you the hand that moves all these things around and places them into constellations? Well, I think you've probably tried to be. You've tried to control, and manipulate, and move these things so that they go in places that you want them to be. Check in with your experience and ask yourself if that's been possible. How has it worked when you've done that?

My guess is that overall, it hasn't worked. I don't know of anyone who has actually been able to order their life quite like that in the long term. So, if you're not the constellations or the stars, and you're not the hand that moves them around, what else could you be?

What if you're the surface on which these things stand? Notice that the surface that you've placed these items upon is metaphorically like the night sky. Consider all this space around and between the stars and the planets – what if that's like you?

It contains all these experiences. It's in contact with all these experiences. And yet, does the surface that they sit upon have control over all of this psychological stuff that happens in life? Probably not.

Similarly, think about it from the perspective of the universe. Does the space around the planets care how they move? Probably not. And yet it's in contact with them.

So just like the surface and the space, there is part of you that is larger than the things you experience – that has been there right through your life and will be with you for ever. This is the part of you that you know as you. Connecting with this part that's larger than all the parts it contains can often allow us to distance ourselves from our issues. It allows us to be a little bit kinder to ourselves, to let go of some of this endless fighting that often ends up causing us more trouble.

So to help you have a visual representation of this, let's come back to the stars you have laid out in front of you. Find that plastic bottle and pop all the items into the bottle – all the items you've attached to yourself to represent the pain, and all the strategies you've attached to yourself. Put some water in it. Put the lid on tightly and maybe put some duct tape around the top of it.

Congratulations, you've made a shaker for your baby!

If your baby's the right age to hold onto it and move it around, give it to them and see what happens. Notice how those different parts all move together. Notice the medium that they're in – the water inside that shaker contains them all, at the same time as being in contact with them all. It contains the different parts, but it isn't defined by them.

Each time you see this shaker and give it to your baby to play with, you can think to yourself, *I'm more than just my pain. There are all these different parts of me, and I can accept them all for what they are.*

SECTION 10

MAKING YOUR MOVE AGAIN, AND AGAIN, AND AGAIN

In the last chapter, you found a space from which to move and begin doing things to take you in the direction of what you really care about. Next, here's an opportunity to learn some more structure around this. You will have the chance to address the things that cause you pain, and reduce your suffering in the longer term. You will start to build patterns that take you towards what you really care about in life.

Firstly, identify the values that you most want to work on right now. It might be that you want to turn back to Section 5 and take another look at your sun diagram. Think about the things in there that you notice were most lacking – in other words, the values that you've done the least work towards. Or it could be that you've got an area of your life that you're really keen to work on. In that case, you can choose the values from that area. Or it might be about something to do with parenting ...

Whatever it is, identify the value that you want to work towards and begin by breaking it down to find a goal that you think is realistic.

It can be helpful here to get a really clear idea of what you want. Ask yourself: *How would I know if this problem was solved? What would I be doing differently?* To help you get really clear on this, you can almost imagine that a film crew is trailing you for a reality TV show. What do you think the viewer of that show would notice that was different? This can give you a good idea of the objective you want to work towards. It can also help you identify other goals further along the way.

If that doesn't help, imagine instead that you have a magic wand and if you wave it, everything will be sorted. Think about that – try to identify three things that would be different about your life if that magic could happen.

Secondly, break your goal down into smaller steps. Notice what the smallest parts of the task are, and allocate a specific length of time each day to work on it. For example, in writing this book, I've been aiming to do ten minutes' work on it every day. Realistically, that became about thirty minutes a week. However, beginning that pattern is part of the key. Find a space that you might be able to allocate to this in your day. Remember that old saying – no one eats an elephant in one sitting! So start small.

Sometimes getting somebody to help you can be useful. Tell other people what your goal is, or get a trusted friend to support you. This is a bit like a journey of a thousand miles starting with just one step. Small but consistent action is often the best way to begin.

Now, do some thinking about where you might need help. Where do you think you'll encounter barriers? How will you manage the logistics? Is this something you know how to do already? Or is one of your goals along the way going to be to learn or acquire new skills? Identify your support crew. And don't forget to build some breaks into your schedule. For example, if you're starting an exercise programme, you need rest days. Make every fourth or fifth day a rest day. Give yourself opportunities for catch up if you need to.

Remember that confidence scale? Start small and get yourself up to seven out of ten on the confidence scale. If you can't get that high, you need to revise down to make the task a little easier. Our goal here is to build patterns of doing new things, and of living in a way that takes you towards things you really care about.

As you get started it can be helpful to tie your activity to a cue or a habit that already exists in your life. For example, if you want to build a pattern to be more mindful, you might choose to do that whenever you get in your car, go to the shops, or take a shower. Or you could set an alarm reminder on your phone so that you get used to taking five or ten minutes for this every day.

If you're working towards a goal of health and wellbeing, you might attach it to a cue of taking a vitamin or brushing your teeth – something you already do every day. For example, I like to drop into the present when I walk my dog every day. Whatever you choose, you can use that as an opportunity to review how well the change you're making is going.

Remember we talked about telling other people about your goals? It can be a partner, a close friend or a relative. And it can be really helpful to ask them to "touch base" with you about how you're getting on with your committed action. If you're really,

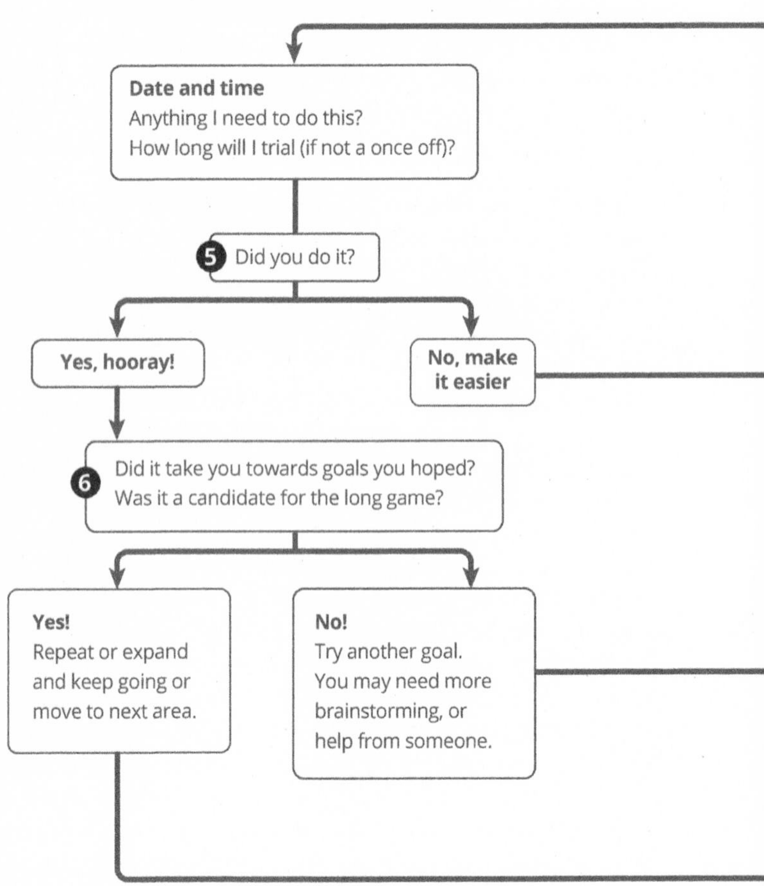

Figure 12: *Committed Action Flow Chart.*

truly committed, you can even share it on social media and ask people to prompt you. At the other end of the scale, you don't even have to tell the person what it is that you're doing if you choose not to. You can just say you're trying out a new habit and you'd love them to ask you how it's going every now and then.

On the next page is a flowchart that summarises the steps we've talked about so that you can begin your own planning.

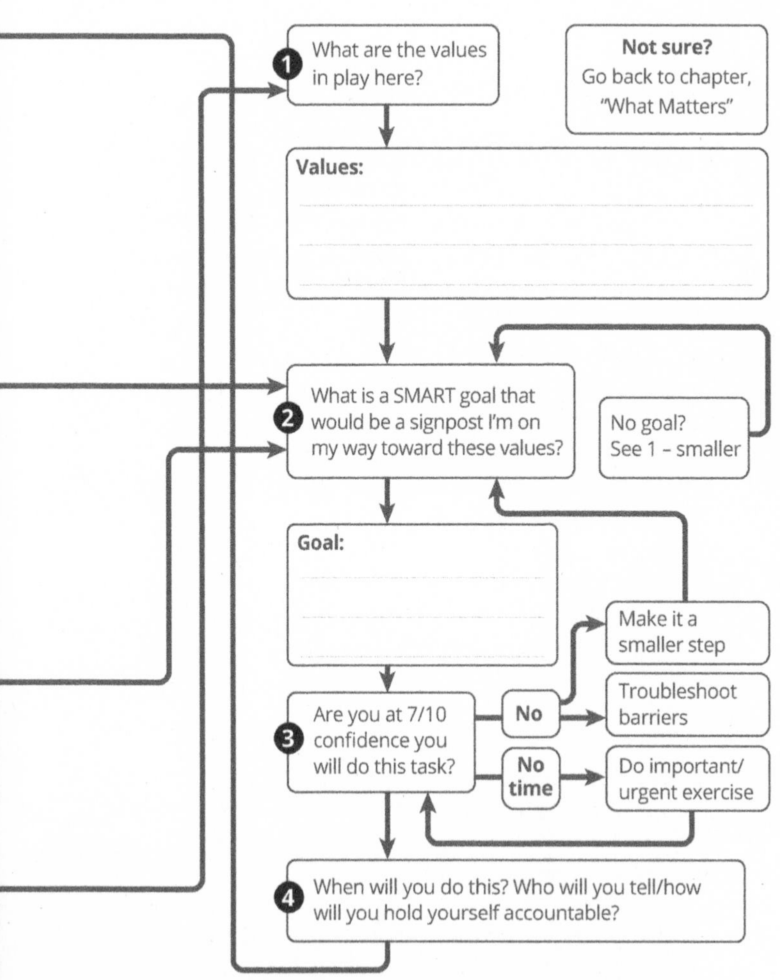

What things might you work on? Here are some examples of kinds of committed action:

1. Learning new skills, e.g. learning to tolerate distress, reading your baby's cues, getting good at noticing patterns in your mind, learning how to care for yourself.
2. Problem-solving.
3. Deliberately putting yourself into anxiety-provoking situations and learning that you can manage them by starting easy and building up to the things that are most scary for you. This would involve putting into practice a whole heap of skills that you've already learnt in this book.
4. Getting your life more consistent with the things that you care about at the level of the activities you do during the day. This could be figuring out the important things that you really want to spend time on, versus the things that just seem important that you would like to de-prioritise.
5. Scheduling pleasant events for yourself, and learning to get out there and do more things. You can also give yourself the chance to once again do the things that you once enjoyed, that gave a sense of meaning to your life. At first, you might have to do things because you've scheduled them rather than because you're enjoying them. You would then go through and rate how much you enjoyed them, or how much of a sense of achievement those events gave you. You'll need to go on doing them and noticing your responses; in time you will probably discover that you start to enjoy yourself more again.

So the great news is that there are lots of resources out there for committed action, and you might be able to find one that really works for you. If there are skills you want to learn, the internet is an amazing resource. You might also be able to find opportunities in your community. Or you may find that you've got enough information here to get started on your own committed action.

Here are some examples of where Sonya undertook committed action. Sonya started learning to do things that she felt anxious about. She undertook a behavioural activation programme with a weekly planner. She scrapbooked, went on walks, and scheduled evenings out with Devon. She worked really coherently and consistently on a pattern for establishing Jack's sleeping and waking cycles during the day and overnight.

One of the other things that Sonya did was learn to make friends with her anxiety and to accept this emotion whenever it came up.

She did a "physicalising" exercise, a type of exercise which I'll share with you shortly. Sonya physicalised the emotions she felt alongside the thoughts of *What if he dies?* She did this in order to be more connected and more able to engage, trust and fully love Jack.

Doing some therapy work is another form of committed action. For example, you read that Sonya did some mother / infant work with Gill, and in the process learnt more about Jack in order to create more of a bond with him.

From the outset, every single one of these things seemed amorphous and huge and beyond her ability. But breaking it down into smaller pieces, identifying the things that she could do, and recognising the small places that she could start, allowed her to begin her journey towards healing.

While there are many places where you can find information about taking committed action, there are some things that our society isn't so good at helping us with. One of these is actually allowing things to be and engaging in willingness and acceptance – especially when it comes to things that we can't change – such as things that are part of us or part of the situation that we live in.

Let me give you some examples of how to take committed action:

PHYSICALISING

As I mentioned, my favourite exercise for committed action with emotions is called physicalising or objectifying (Hayes, 2005). It's about giving a physical form to the experience you're having. There are lots of ways you can do this: you can do it with pens and paper or plasticine. Or you can do it in your mind. I'll give you the steps to do this exercise as if you're doing it with paper and wide range of pastel colours, and then you can vary it and do it in the way that you choose.

Start by identifying the thing that you want to work on. You might need to go back and have another look at the flowchart to help you find something that's the right sort of size for you to work on right now. It could even be something as small as a mild frustration, or it could be something as large as the grief that you feel when you look at your baby and realise that you've lost time with them while you were feeling low.

Start by really becoming present and really noticing this target that you've got. Notice where it is in your body, notice where the edges are, imagine how large it might be ... See if you can breathe in and around this feeling, so that you really notice it. Now, imagine if this feeling could have a colour. Which colour would you choose?

If this feeling were a shape, or marks on the page, what would that look like? Begin drawing ... You might have an idea already, or it might come to you as you begin drawing. What kind of texture does this feeling have? You might need to scratch the pastel or make different kinds of marks to help make the texture on the page.

How large is this feeling? Does it need to take up a large part of the paper? Or is it small and just in the corner? Either is fine. Just notice, right now, how big that feeling is for you.

Are there any other colours involved in this feeling? Are there symbols and thoughts from your memory? Keep working on this drawing until you feel you've captured at least some of what you're feeling inside of you.

Maybe notice if there is a temperature associated with this feeling and see if you can convey that on your page.

Remember to breathe in around the feeling and notice it as you draw.

Now get another piece of paper. You might have noticed that, as you drew the first picture, another feeling emerged. Maybe it was the sense of not wanting that feeling, or wanting to get rid of it. Put the first drawing to one side and now connect with that feeling of repulsion or not wanting to engage with the first feeling.

Now repeat the exercise. What colour is this "wanting to get rid of it" feeling? What shape? Is it fast or slow? Use your colours to make lines or markings to suggest the speed this feeling might go at. How warm or cool is it? Does it have a texture? How large is it? How much of the page will it take up?

Approach this with a sense of playfulness, if you can. Your art doesn't have to be perfect! Keep drawing until you feel like you've captured the feeling of not wanting the painful sensations or emotions from the first picture.

Now place both those pictures together so that you can see them simultaneously. Take a step back. Allow yourself to look at both of them and see if you can bring yourself to a really mindful space of just observing and noticing your sensations and thoughts as you look at these pictures.

Now, as best you can, bring in your willingness. These feelings – and this sense of not wanting – are a part of you. They're a part of your experience. Can you open the door to them and allow them to be there? Are you willing to welcome them – in the kind of way you might welcome a muddy child coming into your clean house?

Notice that you're looking at these feelings. Remember that observer perspective where you discovered that while these feelings are large, there is a part of you that is larger than all that. You are an entity which contains all of your feelings, like the night sky. There is more to you than just these feelings.

Breathe in. Imagine breathing around the feelings, and notice how space begins to emerge as you do so. And now notice ... has anything changed?

It might have, it might not have. Look at the colours in the first picture – do they need altering in any way? Go ahead and alter them, or even start another picture to notice what that original target feels like. Remember to notice characteristics like shape, colour, size, texture, speed. As you do this, stay aware of what's happening.

Here is an example where I physicalised the anxiety I felt about writing and sharing this book, and then my resistance to feeling this anxiety:

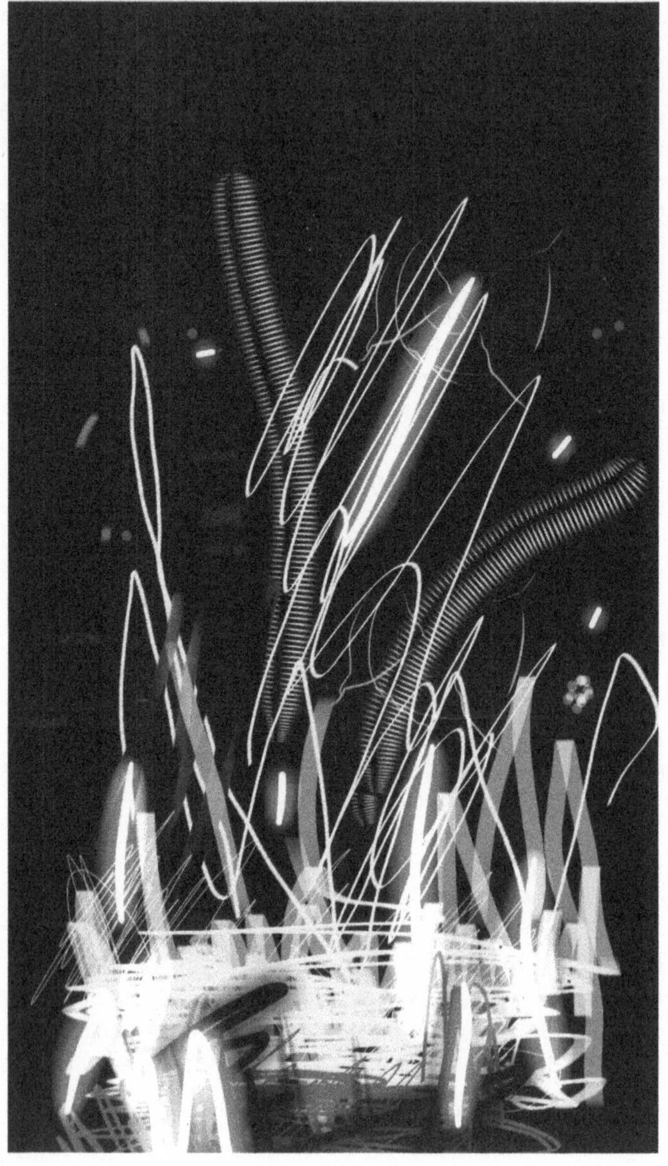

Figure 13: *Kathryn's physicalised anxiety about writing and sharing this book.*

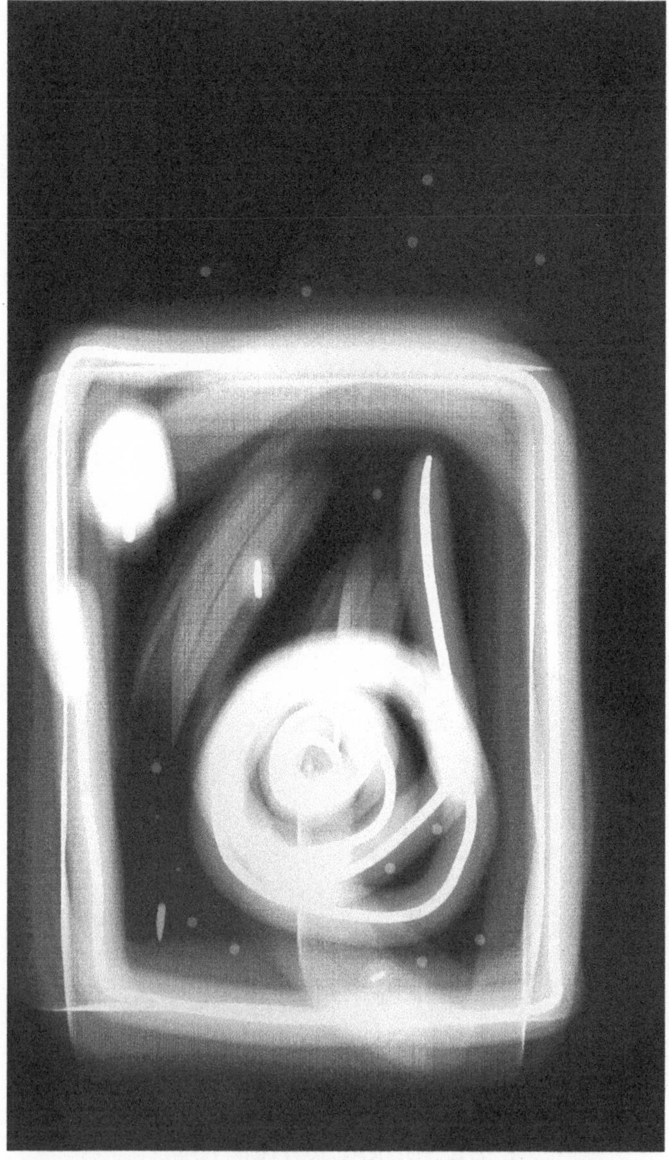

***Figure 14:** Kathryn's physicalised resistance to anxiety about writing and sharing this book.*

To use paints, follow the instructions above, using the fluidity of the paint to help express what you notice even further.

If you want to do this by writing, use words to describe your experiences – you might want to work in a special journal. Make sure you take plenty of time to notice and explore your feelings.

Plasticine allows you to merge colour and shape in a more three-dimensional way and lets you play with surface texture. You might want to incorporate some imagination into how big your physicalised emotions are in real life. Or you can do the emotion and then the resistance in scale with each other.

Now you've finished, you can choose what you do with these pictures. You might like to put them somewhere that you'll notice them as an explicit reminder to practise acceptance and tuning into your feelings. Or you might like to fold them up small and put them somewhere where you'll unintentionally discover them at later point. For example, you could put them in one of your winter boots, in the pocket of a coat you only wear occasionally, or in the side pocket of a bag or backpack.

The purpose of putting away or carrying these pictures / objects / writing is not to hide or get rid of these experiences. It's to allow yourself to carry them with you, or to rediscover them at a future point, so that you can reflect and notice if the experience is still the same for you. Sometimes this can be quite a cathartic exercise and sometimes it can be intense and leave people feeling quite vulnerable.

I'd invite you now to practise taking care of yourself and showing yourself a little bit of kindness if you feel vulnerable after doing this exercise. Identify something that you can do that would help to soothe you. That might be as simple as going to make your favourite hot drink, cuddling up with a pet, or reading something nice. It could be that you need someone to be with you right now. Do whatever you need to do, and as ever, at any point you can choose to stop being willing and see what that's like as well.

ANTI-ROUTINE ROUTINE AND BEHAVIOURAL ACTIVATION

When our mood is low, we often stop doing the things that once caused us to feel good, gave meaning to our lives or gave us a sense of achievement. Once we've withdrawn from these activities, we lose the chance to experience the positive feelings that go along with them. In turn, this can lead to thinking, *There's no point anyway* or *I'll do it when I feel like it*. Uh oh. Vicious cycle ...

A long-established, and still incredibly potent treatment for depression, is called "behavioural activation". It involves identifying what you once enjoyed doing, scheduling these activities into your day, then doing the activities just because they're scheduled (not because you necessarily feel like doing them). Once you've done the activity, you rate how much pleasure and achievement you actually experienced doing them. As you keep doing this over a period of a few weeks, you'll usually discover your ratings for pleasure and achievement increase. There is really good evidence that this intervention works: in fact, it may be the most potent part of CBT (Jacobson et al, 1996). So give it a go!

But hold on! One of the challenges of doing behavioural activation in the perinatal period is that your time is already FULL. You already have a lot of slog and repetitive things that you have to do. Adding more stuff is often the last thing you need. And let's face it, most babies are not really schedule-led creatures, especially early on! So if these kinds of barriers are present for you, here's how I modify behavioural activation for the mums I work with. It's called the anti-routine routine, and it's based around the rhythms and patterns of a day with a baby.

First step, you may need to carve out time. (If you have already have a time you can do this, that's awesome! You get to move forward one step now!) But if you need to identify some time, it will probably mean that you choose to spend less time on something else, do something more efficient, or give up another activity entirely. Eisenhower had a helpful way of identifying where you might find some potential spaces called The Eisenhower Method. Think of the things you do in a day, and sort them into these four quadrants (I've started off with some ideas from my experience as examples; if they don't fit for you, just cross them out!):

Important and Urgent ***DO: do it now*** Feed the baby when she wakes	**Important but Not Urgent** ***DECIDE: schedule a time for it*** Blow raspberries on baby's tummy Call up my best friend and natter
Urgent but Not Important ***DELEGATE OR DECIDE: who else could do it? Do I actually need to do it? If necessary, schedule as low priority*** Wash the nappies Answer the phone straight away	**Neither Urgent nor Important** ***ELIMINATE: don't do it at all or postpone indefinitely*** Do the vacuuming again so big kids can traipse mud through the house this afternoon Tidy out drawers

Figure 15: *The Eisenhower Method showing the things you do in a day, with examples from Kathryn's experience.*

OR:

The Eisenhower Box

	URGENT	NOT URGENT
IMPORTANT	**DO** ***Do it now.*** Write article for today.	**Decide** ***Schedule a time to do it.*** Exercising. Calling family and friends. Researching articles. Long-term biz strategy.
NOT IMPORTANT	**Delegate** ***Who can do it for you?*** Scheduling interviews. Booking flights. Approving comments. Answering certain emails. Sharing articles.	**Delete** ***Eliminate it.*** Watching television. Checking social media. Sorting through junk mail.

What is important is seldom urgent and what is urgent is seldom important.
Dwight Eisenhower, 34th President of the United States.

Figure 16: *The Eisenhower Box.*

Okay, so what was in the bottom row for you? Especially in the Not Urgent Nor Important category? Those are the things that you could consider for deletion, delay or outsourcing. Would you be willing to vacuum less often to give yourself time to do something for your health? Could you employ a nappy service to do the washing? Is it time to bank in all those offers of meals from friends and family, or do a really lazy dinner to give yourself an extra fifteen minutes to look after your own needs? It might help you be more sustainable long-term.

This process will involve trade-offs. Use your acceptance skills here, keep practising letting go and play the long-term game. Personally, I'm still working on accepting mess around the house in service of time to sit down and rest (ask my partner) and I have discovered this makes me a much nicer mother to be around. It helps me keep going in the long term.

Okay, now you've got at least some time. Start by brainstorming or identifying the things you currently or previously enjoyed doing, or got a sense of achievement from. If you want to get really organised about this, check out the pleasant events schedule below by Linehan, 1993. Highlight the things that are possible in the time you have. You may need to get creative here, seek help, or consider babysitting options).

PLEASANT EVENTS SCALE

On the next page is a list of events that many people enjoy, find pleasant or gain a sense of achievement from. Rate each event for BOTH enjoyment (E) and achievement (A) on a scale of 1 – 10, where:

1 = I hate doing this / no achievement at all

5 = Medium enjoyment / achievement

10 = I love doing this / it gives me a sense of massive achievement.

E	A	
		1. Soaking in the bathtub
		2. Planning my career
		3. Getting out of (paying off) debt
		4. Collecting things (coins, etc.)
		5. Going on vacation
		6. Thinking how it will be when I finish school
		7. Recycling old items
		8. Going on a date
		9. Relaxing
		10. Going to a movie in the middle of the week
		11. Jogging, walking
		12. Thinking I have done a full day's work
		13. Listening to music
		14. Recalling past parties
		15. Buying household gadgets
		16. Lying in the sun
		17. Planning a career change
		18. Laughing
		19. Thinking about my past trips
		20. Listening to others
		21. Reading magazines or newspapers
		22. Hobbies (stamp collecting, model building, etc.)
		23. Spending an evening with good friends
		24. Planning a day's activities
		25. Meeting new people
		26. Remembering beautiful scenery

E	A	
		27. Saving money
		28. Gambling
		29. Going home from work
		30. Eating
		31. Practising karate, judo, or yoga
		32. Thinking about retirement
		33. Repairing things around the house
		34. Working on my car or bicycle
		35. Remembering the words and deeds of loving people
		36. Wearing sexy clothes
		37. Having quiet evenings
		38. Taking care of my plants
		39. Buying, selling stock
		40. Going swimming
		41. Doodling
		42. Exercising
		43. Collecting old things
		44. Going to a party
		45. Thinking about buying things
		46. Playing golf
		47. Playing soccer
		48. Flying kites
		49. Having discussions with friends
		50. Having family get-togethers
		51. Riding a motorbike
		52. Sex

E	A	
		53. Running track
		54. Going camping
		55. Singing around the house
		56. Arranging flowers
		57. Practising religion (going to church, group praying, etc.)
		58. Losing weight
		59. Going to the beach
		60. Thinking I'm an okay person
		61. A day with nothing to do
		62. Having class reunions
		63. Going skating
		64. Going sailboating
		65. Traveling abroad or in N.Z.
		66. Painting
		67. Doing something spontaneously
		68. Doing needlepoint, crewel, etc.
		69. Sleeping
		70. Driving
		71. Entertaining
		72. Going to clubs (youth group, music group etc.)
		73. Thinking about getting married
		74. Going hunting
		75. Singing with groups
		76. Flirting
		77. Playing musical instrument
		78. Doing arts and crafts

E	A	
		79. Making a gift for someone
		80. Buying records
		81. Watching boxing, wrestling
		82. Planning parties
		83. Cooking
		84. Going hiking
		85. Writing books (poems, articles)
		86. Sewing
		87. Buying clothes
		88. Going out to dinner
		89. Working
		90. Discussing books
		91. Sightseeing
		92. Gardening
		93. Going to the beauty parlour
		94. Early-morning coffee and newspaper
		95. Playing tennis
		96. Kissing
		97. Watching children (play)
		98. Thinking I have a lot more going for me than most people
		99. Going to plays and concerts
		100. Daydreaming
		101. Planning to go to school
		102. Thinking about sex
		103. Going for a drive
		104. Listening to a stereo

E	A	
		105. Refinishing furniture
		106. Watching TV
		107. Making lists of tasks
		108. Going bike riding
		109. Walks in the woods (or at the waterfront)
		110. Buying gifts
		111. Traveling to national parks
		112. Completing a task
		113. Collecting shells
		114. Going to a spectator sport (auto racing, horse racing)
		115. Eating gooey, fattening foods
		116. Teaching
		117. Photography
		118. Going fishing
		119. Thinking about pleasant events
		120. Staying on a diet
		121. Playing with animals
		122. Flying a plane
		123. Reading fiction
		124. Acting
		125. Being alone
		126. Writing diary entries or letters
		127. Cleaning
		128. Reading nonfiction
		129. Taking children places
		130. Dancing

E	A	
		131. Going on a picnic
		132. Thinking I did that pretty well after doing something
		133. Meditating
		134. Playing volleyball
		135. Having lunch with a friend
		136. Going to the mountains
		137. Thinking about having a family
		138. Thoughts about happy moments in my childhood
		139. Splurging
		140. Playing cards
		141. Solving riddles mentally
		142. Having a political discussion
		143. Playing softball
		144. Seeing and / or showing photos or slides
		145. Playing guitar
		146. Knitting
		147. Doing crossword puzzles
		148. Shooting pool
		149. Dressing up and looking nice
		150. Reflecting on how I've improved
		151. Buying things for myself (perfume, golf balls, etc.)
		152. Talking on the phone
		153. Going to museums
		154. Thinking religious thoughts
		155. Lighting candles
		156. Listening to the radio

E	A	
		157. Getting a massage
		158. Saying 'I love you'
		159. Thinking about my good qualities
		160. Buying books
		161. Taking a sauna or a steam bath
		162. Going skiing
		163. White-water canoeing
		164. Going bowling
		165. Doing woodworking
		166. Fantasising about the future
		167. Taking ballet, tap dancing
		168. Debating
		169. Sitting in a sidewalk café
		170. Having an aquarium
		171. Erotica (sex books, movies)
		172. Going horseback riding
		173. Thinking about becoming active in the community
		174. Doing something new
		175. Making jigsaw puzzles
		176. Thinking I'm a person who can cope
		177. Walking the dog
		178. Playing the piano

Figure 17: *Pleasant Events Scale.*

Now use the anti-routine routine to schedule your activity. Try to get yourself to 7 / 10 confidence. But if you can't make 7 / 10, break it down into something smaller. Ideally, do at least one activity a day, using the ideas above to help you to remember to do the thing you've scheduled. Stick your routine up on the fridge or somewhere you'll see it. How long will you commit to doing this for? What values does it connect with? Consider giving yourself a reward you'll enjoy for each week you keep it up (sounds corny, but it does actually work)!

THE ANTI-PLAN PLANNER FOR SCHEDULING AND GOING WITH THE FLOW

Use the planner on the next page to help you schedule things that give you a sense of enjoyment or achievement, around the (often) unpredictable needs of a baby. If your baby does regularly sleep during the day, note those times in as well on the "rhythm" column.

Rhythm	Monday	Tuesday	Wednesday	Thursday	Friday	Saturday	Sunday
Waking							
Breakfast							
Lunch							
Dinner							
Bedtime							
Overnight							

THE ANTI-TIME TABLE: GO WITH THE FLOW PLANNER

Use this planner to help you figure out things to do around your baby's rhythm for the day. Begin by noting in any points when your baby regularly sleeps, if they do so. You can also use this planner to help you identify where you might need help or support.

Day & Date Today:	Notes, Ideas, Requests
Wake Up	
Breakfast	
Lunch	
Dinner	
Bedtime	

Here's an example for someone's day. They've written their baby's rhythm in bold, then planned around this.

Day and Date Today: *Monday 5th March*	Notes, Ideas, Requests
Wake Up	
Pump and clean bottles *Dad feeds baby breakfast*	
Breakfast	
Floor time playing together *Baby sleeps for half an hour (if I'm lucky ...)* *Spend a long time feeding baby*	*Do some relaxation to get ready for the long feed? Defuse from thoughts about unending nature of feeding.*
Lunch	
Walk? *Baby sleeps then wakes up REALLY grumpy* *Best friend visits on the way home from work and helps me make dinner*	*Have a nap yourself* *Go for a walk to soothe yourself and baby*
Dinner	
Bath time for baby – best time for giggles :) *Baby goes to bed – read a story first* *ME TIME – watch something funny (Dad goes up to soothe baby if she wakes)*	*Maybe get some more books from the library so I've got more variety?*

Just do it! And once it's done, rate how much enjoyment and achievement you got from this activity. Review after a week and tweak the schedule as needed. You may need to do some problem-solving or make the activities easier if you found you weren't doing what you planned. If you got going and kept going, hooray! Well done, you. I hope it's taking you closer and closer towards what truly matters for you.

CONCLUSION

When I first met Sonya, she was a dishevelled, exhausted-looking woman. She was still smiling and pushing baby Jack around in a pushchair, because he was too heavy to carry around the ward. But she looked like she had the weight of the world on her shoulders. Now that you've read her story, you can understand why.

Eight years later, I met Sonya again to talk to her about the idea of writing this book. She was smiling, made-up, bouncy, and her hair was in its usual top knot. The smile that she gave me was so broad – and so genuine – that it became immediately clear to me the difference between the mask that Sonya had worn when she was depressed and this real Sonya that I was seeing in front of me now. She was enthused, eager, keen to get started, and full of ideas.

Hold onto this picture of Sonya – this is a picture of hope for you too. When you come through this, you might discover that you've grown in all sorts of new and interesting ways that you could never have predicted prior to having children and / or becoming depressed.

As you've worked through this book, you will have had the opportunity to learn how to become more aware, more open and more engaged in your life. Are you the kind of person who gets annoyed at red lights? I had a suspicion that Sonya might be. And there's something incredibly useful here: the idea of being open, aware, and engaged maps nicely onto a set of traffic lights. The red light is a pause – a chance to stop, notice, and become aware. Opening up is like the amber light, as you get ready to go, giving yourself the chance to engage with new possibilities. Opening up to accept what is here so that you can respond to the green light is like getting going and moving your life forward. It's all about engaging in discovering what it is that matters to you. It's about taking action, even if it's just a tiny step forward at first.

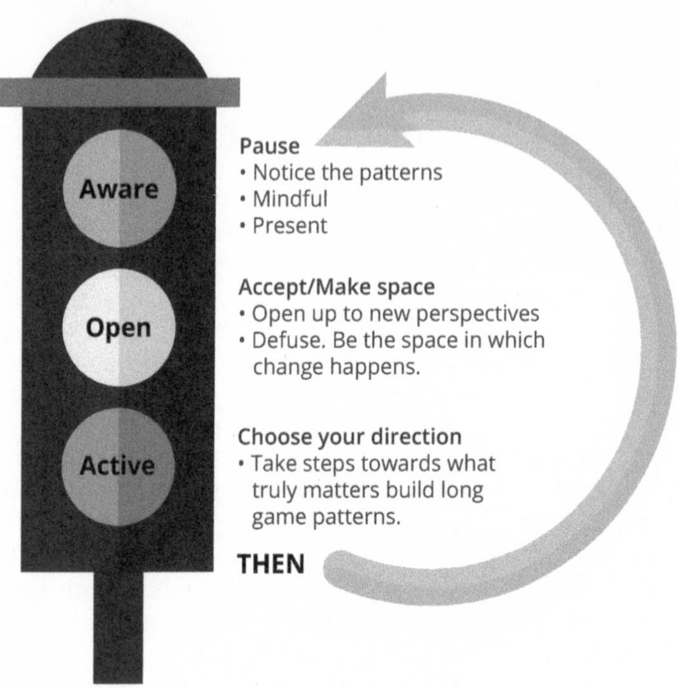
Aware
Open
Active
Pause
• Notice the patterns
• Mindful
• Present
Accept/Make space
• Open up to new perspectives
• Defuse. Be the space in which change happens.
Choose your direction
• Take steps towards what truly matters build long game patterns.
THEN

Figure 18: *Illustration of Aware, Open and Engaged (phrase from Hayes, Villatte, Levin and Hildebrandt, 2011).*

ARE YOU READY?

As you move, you'll probably discover that you encounter new varieties of the pains that maybe led you to pick up this book in the first place.

One of the things that you might take away from this experience is the feeling that you are struggling less. You might have the discovery that, as you let go, you no longer have to fight these things that hurt you. As you make room for them, so too the space in which you live can grow.

At the outset, how much of the time were you trying to cut out some of the experiences that you struggled to deal with? How often did you have feelings of anxiety, feelings of low mood, wishing that the days before you had a baby could come back?

How often did it feel like it was possible to carve yourself up into little pieces and still be alive?

And now, is there more room for those things? Are those things allowed to come with you as you carry on doing what truly matters to you? And as you do so, you'll discover that you re-encounter new things that will challenge you.

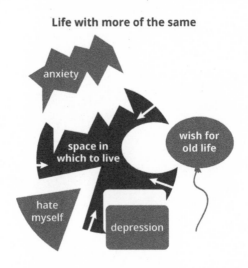

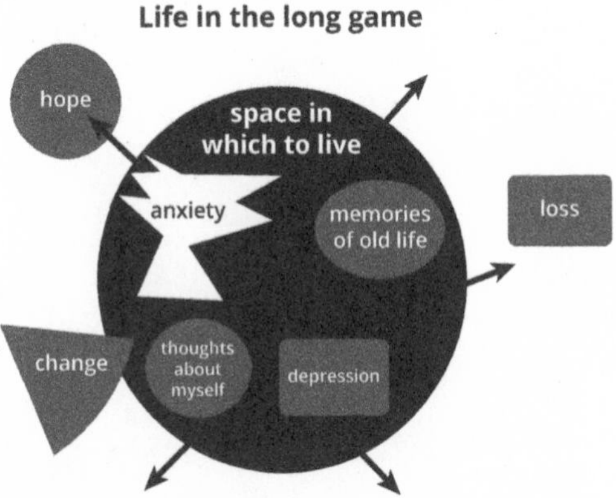

Figure 19: *Life in the Long Game.*

Congratulations! You have started on a journey that just keeps going, and gets bigger and wider and opens up more possibilities and more hope. There's no magic wand here, but I can promise you that things will change, and they can certainly get better. You now have the opportunity to choose to respond to those changes in a way that helps you in the long game.

I wish you all the best on your journey.

RECOMMENDED RESOURCES

- www.mothersmatter.co.nz
- Naomi Stadlen (2004): *What Mothers Do: especially when it looks like they're doing nothing*. Piatkus.
- Daniel Siegel and Mary Hartzell (2013): *Parenting from the Inside Out: How a Deeper Self-Understanding Can Help You Raise Children Who Thrive*. Penguin USA.
- Kathryn Black (2005) *Mothering Without a Map: The Search for the Good Mother within*. Penguin.
- Lynne Murray and Liz Andrews (2001): *Your Social Baby: Understanding Babies' Communication from Birth*. Australian Council of Educational Research.
- Margot Sunderland (2016): *The Science of Parenting* (2nd ed). Dorling Kindersley.
- Koa Whittingham (2013): *Becoming Mum*. Pivotal Publishing. www.koawhittingham.com
- Russ Harris (2007 and 2012): *The Happiness Trap and The Reality Slap*. Robinson.
- Steven Hayes (2005) *Get Out of Your Mind and Into Your Life*. New Harbinger.
- www.contextualscience.org/act_for_the_public

REFERENCES

Ashman S.B. & Dawson, G. (2012). *Maternal depression, infant psychobiological development, and risk for depression in children of depressed parents: Mechanisms of risk and implications for treatment.* Goodman, S.H. & Gotlib I.H. (Eds.) Washington, DC: American Psychological Association.

Baur A., Parsonage M., Knapp M., Lemmi V. & Adelaja B. (Oct 2014). *The costs of perinatal health problems.* Centre for Mental Health and Personal Social Services Research Unit.

Bennett I.M., Marcus S.C., Palmer S.C. & Coyne J.C. (2010). *Pregnancy-related discontinuation of antidepressants and depression care visits among Medicaid recipients.* Psychiatric Services. 61(4):386–91.

Bergener, Monk, Werner. (2008). *Dyadic intervention during pregnancy? Treating pregnant women and possibly reaching the future baby.* Infant Mental Health Journal. 29(5):399–419.

Biaggi A., Conroy S., Pawlby S. & Pariante C. M. (2016). *Identifying the women at risk of antenatal anxiety and depression: a systematic review.* Journal of affective disorders. 191, 62–77.

Bledsoe S. & Grote N. (2006). *Treating depression during pregnancy and the postpartum: a preliminary meta-analysis.* Research on Social Work Practice. 16, 109–20.

Cooper P. J., Murray L., Wilson A. & Romaniuk H. (2003). *Controlled trial of the short-and long-term effect of psychological treatment of post-partum depression.* The British Journal of Psychiatry. 182(5), 412–19.

Cox J.L., Holden J.M. & Sagovsky, R. (1987). *Detection of postnatal depression: Development of the 10-item Edinburgh Postnatal Depression Scale.* British Journal of Psychiatry. 150:782–86.

Dennis C. L. & Dowswell, T. (2013). *Psychosocial and psychological interventions for preventing postpartum depression.*

The Cochrane Library.
Dunkel Schetter C. (2011). *Psychological science on pregnancy: Stress processes, biopsychosocial models, and emerging research issues*. Annual Review of Psychology. 62, 531–58.
Dunkel Schetter C. & Tanner L. (2012). *Anxiety, depression and stress in pregnancy: implications for mothers, children, research, and practise*. Current Opinion in Psychiatry. 25(2), 141–8.
Dahl J. & Lundgren T. (2006). *Living beyond your pain: Using Acceptance and Commitment Therapy to ease chronic pain*. Oakland, California: New Harbinger.
Dennis C. L. & Dowswell T. (2013). *Psychosocial and psychological interventions for preventing postpartum depression*. The Cochrane Library.
'Eisenhower Method' in Wikipedia 'Time Management' Retrieved from: https://en.wikipedia.org/wiki/Time_management. 05/07/2019.
Glover V. (2014). *Maternal depression, anxiety and stress during pregnancy and child outcome; what needs to be done*. Best Practice & Research Clinical Obstetrics and Gynaecology. 28(1), 25–35.
Hayes S.C. (2005). *Get out of your mind and into your life*. Oakland, California: New Harbinger.
Hayes S.C., Villatte M., Levin M. & Hildebrandt M. (2011). *'Open, aware and active: contextual approaches as an emerging trend in the behavioral and cognitive therapies'*. Annual Review of Clinical Psychology. Vol 7,141–68.
Hayes S.C., Barnes-Holmes D., Roche B., eds (2001). *Relational frame theory: A post-Skinnerian account of human language and cognition*. New York: Kluwer Academic / Plenum.
Hayes S.C., Strosahl K.D. & Wilson K.G. (2012). *Acceptance and commitment therapy: The process and practice of mindful change*. (2nd edition). Oakford, CA: New Harbinger.
Hinton L., Bavetta M., Robinson J., Kenyon S., Knight M. & Kurinczuk J. (2015). *Saving Lives, Improving Mother's Care 2015: Lay Report*. Mothers and Babies: Reducing Risk through audits and confidential enquires across the UK. (MBRRACE-UK).
Linehan M.M. (1993). *Skills Training Manual for Treating Borderline Personality Disorder*. New York: Guildford Press.

Jacobson N.Z., Dobson K.S., Truax P.A., Addis M.E., Koerner K., Gollan J.K., Gortner E. & Price S.E. (1996). *A component analysis of cognitive behavioural treatment for depression*. Journal of Consulting and Clinical Psychology. 64(2).

Knight M., et al. (2014). *Saving Lives, Improving Mothers' Care – Lessons learned to inform future maternity care from the UK and Ireland Confidential Enquiries into Maternal Deaths and Morbidity 2009–2012*. Oxford: University of Oxford.

Martins C. & Gaffan E. A. (2000). *Effects of early maternal depression on patterns of infant-mother attachment: a meta-analytic investigation*. Journal of Child Psychology and Psychiatry. 41(6), 737–46.

National Institute for Health and Clinical Excellence. (2014). Antenatal and postnatal mental health: *The NICE Guideline on clinical management and service guidance*. Available at: http://www.nice.org.uk/guidance/cg192. 05/07/2019.

O'Hara M.W. & McCabe J.E. *Postpartum depression: current status and future directions*. Annu Rev Clin Psychol. 2013;9:379–407. doi: 10.1146/annurev-clinpsy-050212-185612.

Paulson J.F. & Bazemore S.D. (2010). *Prenatal and postpartum depression in fathers and its association with maternal depression: A meta-analysis. Journal of the American Medical Association*. Vol 303 (19).

Perinatal Mental Health Alliance. (2014). *Call to act.* Available at: http://everyonesbusiness.org.uk/wp-content/uploads/2014/07/Call-to-ACT.pdf.

Perinatal Mental Health Alliance. (2015). *Falling through the gaps: perinatal mental health and general practice*. Available from: http://everyonesbusiness.org.uk/wp-content/uploads/2015/04/RCGP-Report-Falling-through-the-gaps-PMH-and-general-practice-March-2015.pdf. 05/07/2019.

PMMRC. (2015). *Ninth Annual Report of the Perinatal and Maternal Mortality Review Committee: Reporting mortality 2013*. Wellington: Health Quality & Safety Commission.

Primary Care Screening for and Treatment of Depression in Pregnant and Postpartum Women. (2015). *Evidence Report and Systematic Review for the US Preventive Services Task Force*. O'Connor et al. JAMA. 2016;315(4):388–406. doi:10.1001/jama.18948.

Ramchandani et al 2008. *The effects of pre and postnatal depression in fathers: a natural experiment comparing the effects of exposure to depression on offspring*. J. CHILD Psychol Psychiatry, Oct;49(10):1069–78.

Reichenbaum M.E., Moraes C.L., Oliveira A.S.D. & Lobato G. (2011). *Edinburgh postnatal depression scale (EPDS): empirical evidence for a general factor*. BMC Medical Research Methodology.11:93.

Robertson E., Grace S., Wallington T. & Stewart D. E. (2004). *Antenatal risk factors for postpartum depression: a synthesis of recent literature*. General hospital psychiatry. 26(4), 289–95.

Robinson P.J., Gould D.A. & Strosahl K.D. (2011). *Real Behavior Change in Primary Care: Improving patient outcomes and increasing job satisfaction*. New Harbinger: Oakford.

Simms L.J., Gros D.F., Watson D. & O'Hara M.W. (2008). *Parsing the general and specific components of depression and anxiety with bifactor modeling*. Depression and Anxiety. Vol 25: E34-46. 10.1002/da.20432.

Siegel D.J. (1999). *The developing mind: How relationships and the brain interact to shape who we are*. New York: Guilford Press.

Sockol L.E. (2015). *A systematic review of the efficacy of cognitive behavioral therapy for treating and preventing perinatal depression*. Journal of affective disorders. 177, 7–21.

Swain A.M., Ohara M.W., Starr K.R. & Gorman L.L. (1997) *A prospective study of sleep, mood, and cognitive function in postpartum and non-postpartum women*. Obstet Gynaecol90(3): 381–86.

Villatte M., Villatte J.L. & Hayes S.C. (2016). Mastering the Clinical Conversation: *Language as intervention*. New York: Guildford.

Yonkers K.A., Blackwell K.A., Glover J. & Forray A. (2014). *Antidepressant use in pregnant and postpartum women*. Annu Rev Clin Psychol. 10:369–92. doi: 10.1146/annurev-clinpsy-032813-153626. http://europepmc.org/abstract/MED/24313569.

Wisner K.L., Sit D.K., McShea M.C., et al. (2013). *Onset timing, thoughts of self-harm, and diagnoses in postpartum women with screen-positive depression findings*. JAMA Psychiatry; 70: 490–8.

Winnicott D.W. (1964). *The child, the family and the outside world*. Middlesex, England: Penguin.

KATHRYN'S ACKNOWLEDGMENTS

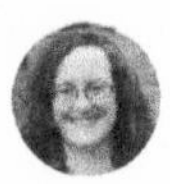

Thank you to Lucas, my hilarious, smart, independent and brave boy, who has taught me far more than I ever expected to learn as a mother.

To Julie for being there. Always.

Thank you to my own mother, Patricia, for inculcating in me the worth of the mothering role, giving me an amazing role model to aspire to and being such a wonderful gran. Thank you to my family and my siblings for putting up with my bossy, oldest-sister mothering.

To my work "mothers", the supervisors and clinicians who have help me grow along the way. A special thank you to Fiona Will, Jackie Donaldson, Liz MacDonald and the rest of the amazing team at the mothers and babies service at CDHB. Nga mihi nui ki a Donna Roberts mo te tautoko me to matauranga. Thank you to the Otautahi ACT Interest Group. Thank you as well as to Sue Galvin and Annmaree Kingi for turning me into an actual ACT therapist. Thank you to Rich Farmer for suggesting one day I might have a book in me, when the prospect was terrifying and an amazing dream. Also to Clare, Helen and Ros for helping me grow, helping me to be ready, and encouraging me to keep doing my work.

Thank you to Colette for the opportunity to BFF through your mothering journey. Thank you for sharing your beautiful daughter with me, so that I remember the potential of all the babies I see.

And to Sonya and all the mothers I have worked with: thank you for allowing me the privilege of sharing some of your journey along the way, for your patience with me, and all the ways you have shaped me to better understand and serve you.

SONYA'S ACKNOWLEDGMENTS

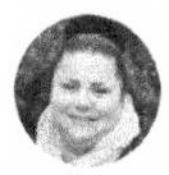

Thank you to my son Jack – if it wasn't for Jack I wouldn't be doing what I'm doing today. I have learnt so much from him and continue to learn daily. He brought out my passion to support other mums.

Thank you to Lily for giving me another chance at motherhood.

To my amazing husband Devon: thank you for loving me, supporting me and holding me. I am truly blessed to have you as my husband, best friend and wonderful father to Jack and Lily.

To my family, thank you for being there for us.

To Nanny Barb, you were a godsend in Blenheim, thank you.

Trudy, my Burnham buddy – thank you for listening and not judging.

To my friend Melissa Kelly, thank you for being a wonderful friend.

To Mark Beales, thank you for supporting Devon.

Thank you, RNZAF, for your ongoing support while Devon was in the Air Force.

Others that have been part of my journey on a professional scale: thank you for everything. I wouldn't be where I am today without your professional support:

Chris Templeton of the Plunket Postnatal Adjustment Programme.

The team at the mothers and babies unit at the Princess Margret Hospital, Christchurch: Kathryn Whitehead, Gill Graham, Katy Brett, Liz MacDonald and Debbie Wilson.

Thanks to the inpatient nurses at mothers and babies at the Princess Margaret Hospital, Christchurch: Christine, Julie, Lynn, Brian, Toni and Judy.

I can't thank you all enough. I survived postnatal depression and I'm here to watch my family grow up – thank you xxx

"Postnatal Depression – a journey no mother should have to travel alone."

INDEX

A

acceptance and commitment therapy
  see ACT
acceptance *vs.* resignation, 140–1
ACT, 72–4, 139
  antenatal depression
  anxiety, 30–1
  Apgar test 26
  controlling instinct, 11–12
  criteria for 117
  C-sections, 23–6
  delayed grief 19
  initial experiences, 6–10
  mix of feelings, 32–3
  pregnancy scans, 15–16
  stress management, 17–22
anti-plan planner, 198–9
anti-routine routine, 190–2
anti-time table, 200–1
anxiety, 30–1
  general risk factors 122
anxiety after childbirth
  experiential avoidance, 120–21
  generalised anxiety disorder 120
  obsessive compulsive disorder 120
  panic attacks 120
Apgar test 26
arousal levels, 99–101
attachment, 125–6
aware, open and engaged illustration 203

B

Beck Depression Inventory 74
behavioural activation, 190–2
bili bed 30
bonding, 125–6
Brett, Katy 60

C

cholinesterase 25
choroid plexus cysts 13
cognitive defusion 155
cognitive diffusion skills 73
cognitive fusion 155
committed action flow chart, 182–5
community support, 84–5
compassion, 37–8
coping strategy, 115–16

D

Dahl, JoAnne 131
defusion, 167–8
delayed grief 19
depression
  characteristics of 117
  Edinburgh Postnatal Depression
Scale, 118–19
  general risk factors 122
  maternal 123
  symptoms 118
  things for society 124
domperidone 39

E

Edinburgh Postnatal Depression Scale
  see EPDS
Edinburgh scale 81
Eisenhower box 193
Eisenhower method 192
emotional wellbeing 98
engaging yourself 102

environmental conditions 96
EPDS, 118–19
experiential avoidance, 120–21

F

flow chart, committed action, 182–5
flow planner, anti-time table, 200–1

G

GAD 120
Gaviscon 39
generalised anxiety disorder see GAD
Get Out of Your Mind and into Your Life: the New Acceptance and Commitment Therapy (Hayes) 139
Graham, Gill 60
guilty feelings, 37–8

H

Hayes, Steve 139

I

ibuprofen 62
instinct, controlling, 11–12

L

lumbar puncture, 64–5
Lundgren, Tobias 131

M

mania 121
maternal depression 123
meningococcal disease, 63–5
metaphors, 103–5
mindfulness
  case example-shiny bottles, 152–4
  of eating chocolates, 142–5
  of feeding baby, 145–8
  flexibly dropping into, 150–2
  of watching baby, 148–150
mindfulness skills 73
mix of feelings, 32–3
mother, experiment with, 161–8

N

narcissists 2
nondeclarative memories 125

O

observer perspective 176
observer stance 73
obsessive compulsive disorder *see* OCD
OCD 120
oxytocin 33

P

pacifiers 104
PAFT 84
Pamol 62
panic attacks 120
parenting, traditional societies 3
Parents as First Teachers *see* PAFT
perinatal, definition of 117
perinatal mental health, 117–26
physicalizing/objectifying, 185–90
pleasant events scale, 193–8
PNAP, 52, 83
Postnatal Adjustment Programme *see* PNAP
postnatal (postpartum) depression
  community support, 84–5
  compassion, 37–8
  criteria for 117
  Edinburgh scale 81
  lack of social support 3
  psychological distress 68
  sleep deprivation, 49–50
pregnancy scans, 15–16
psychological distress 68
psychosis
  definition of 121
  risk time for, 121–2

R

ranitidine 39
relapse prevention 73

resignation *vs.* acceptance, 140–1
rupture and repair process, 1–2

S

safety 97
self-soothing, 99–101
sleep deprivation, 49–50
Sotos syndrome, 53–4
space around yourself, 169–79
expansiveness into action, 173–6
fitting together 171
making move again and again, 180–2
observer perspective 176
things that helps 172
time and 172
"splitter" perspective 121
stress management, 17–22
struggling with yourself, 106–9
sun diagram for values, 130–1

T

trauma, 98–9

U

urinary tract infection *see* UTI
UTI, 39, 44

V

values
recognising your, 131–2
sun diagram for, 130–1
writing steps or action 134
vicious cycle 79
vulnerability 4

W

Whanau New Zealand Trust, 83, 84
Whitehead, Kathryn, 70–1
willingness, 139–40
Winnicott, Donald 1

**If you found this book interesting ...
read this sample chapter next.**

When the Bough Breaks

The Pursuit of Motherhood

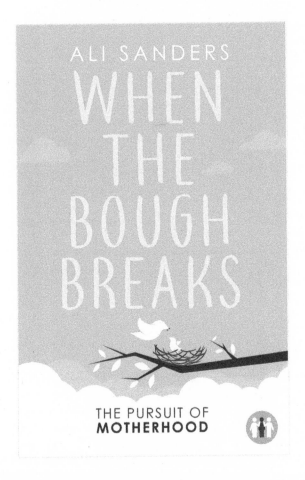

Motherhood was all Ali Sanders had ever wanted out of life.
She just didn't expect it to be such a rocky road to happiness.

EXTRACT FROM WHEN THE BOUGH BREAKS

Fragments

I find it so hard to write this, but I didn't feel a connection to my son when he was born.

What I remember are fragments; parts of the hours and days that followed that fit together but somehow also don't. I remember that Jacob was crying from the shock of being so rudely thrust into the outside world. I remember that as soon as he was placed on my chest, he calmed down. I remember feeling like I was moving around in a daze, as though I was in slow motion and everything else was continuing at normal pace around me.

We were taken into another room where Jacob was weighed and dressed in his tiny first outfit, which was grey and white and said "Little Bear" on the hat. I was able to have a shower. In those few minutes, it was a relief to be away from him for even a few minutes – I instantly hated the notion that he was supposed to be an extension of me in those early days. I just wanted to be autonomous again, to be my own person.

This was so at odds with the mother I'd always thought I would be. I'd always pictured myself with my baby permanently attached to me, day and night. I was going to be a sling-wearing, breastfeeding-on-demand, skin-to-skin earth mother. That was just how it was going to be. So feeling like I wanted to be apart from Jacob so soon after his birth just confused my befuddled mind even more.

After my shower we were shown to a side room which would be our home for the next few hours at least. I needed to go to the toilet, so I left Jacob with Michael while I ensconced myself in the clinical, white bathroom with some magazines that I'd brought along to read while I was waiting for my induction to take effect. (As it happened, I had barely even glanced at them before my labour had begun in earnest.)

I felt incredibly guilty for using the bathroom as a way to be alone; I knew I was expected to be with my baby indefinitely during that time, yet here I was, taking my time and reading magazines while Jacob and Michael were left to it in the other room. As I leafed through the articles, I felt jealous of all the celebrities who were happily living their lives, smiling out from the pages at me. *Would I ever smile again?* I wondered. *Would I ever feel or look like me again?* I didn't understand how all those celebrity mums seemed to be just carrying on as normal, as though they had never even had babies. I looked on in awe at the new mums who were pictured on nights out just days after giving birth – how on earth was that socially acceptable when "ordinary" women like me had it drummed into us that we must not let our babies out of our sights? And how were they not so exhausted that it was all they could do to venture outside to put the bins out, let alone go out into town? As if we don't already put enough pressure on ourselves to be the perfect mum, we also have society's version of perfection thrust upon us as well. And then we sit in universities across the land and wonder why postnatal depression is so prevalent.

*

Once back in the room with Jacob and Michael, I tried my first breastfeed. Other than having seen friends breastfeeding, I had no clue at all what I was supposed to be doing. I put Jacob to the breast; he made some suckling movements, then, a few seconds later, his mouth slipped off again. In my fog of exhaustion, reality was skewed, and I figured that he must have fed for long enough. *Perhaps newborns only need a few seconds per feed*, I thought.

At about nine o'clock, Michael went home. We hadn't been told that he was allowed to stay with us overnight (we only found that bit out later), so I was left alone with Jacob. Each time I laid my head on the pillow to try to rest, he would squirm and cry for another feed. And so the cycle continued throughout the night; a few seconds' worth of feeding followed by two minutes' rest, followed by squirming and crying, followed by another feed. I pressed the buzzer for assistance a couple of times – once because I had passed a huge blood clot that needed to be checked (it turned out to be fine) and once to say that Jacob had passed his first stool. I had been told earlier that I must tell someone when Jacob passed his first bowel movement so it could be checked; however, the nurse that came to me said that wasn't the case and I felt a bit silly for having done so afterwards.

'Everything going alright with the breastfeeding?' she asked, as she turned to leave the room.

'Err ... yes, okay I think.'

I started to explain about the tiny feeds that only lasted for a few seconds at a time, but she had already gone. The staff were very clearly overworked and I felt guilty for bothering them. I assumed they thought that I should know what I was doing at 30 years old and should have been able to look after my baby on my own.

At about four o'clock in the morning, I called for help and told the nurse who came that I was worried I wasn't feeding Jacob properly, as he was only staying latched for a few seconds at a time. She explained that she didn't have time to show me but that she could give me a booklet on breastfeeding to read. I spent the rest of the night trying to work out what the hell I was supposed to be doing, trying to adopt the positions shown in the booklet with Jacob in my arms while being so tired I couldn't see straight. I tried several of the different positions suggested, but there was no improvement in his latch. I felt vulnerable and frightened and couldn't stop shaking. I felt like I was failing my son.

When Michael came back in the morning, I told him about my struggles with the breastfeeding. He went to fetch help and a complete angel of a healthcare assistant came in to spend some time with us. She made me feel human again for a while, talking about her family and her life outside the hospital, and she even managed to make me laugh. She told me about a time when her son had been trying to grow some tomato plants in the garage. She was convinced they needed light, so she moved them onto the kitchen windowsill and started to tend to them. All was fine until her son came home and started to panic, quickly herding his precious plants back into the garage. That was when she realised they weren't tomato plants at all, but cannabis. Up until that point, I'd imagined life had stopped outside the hospital, outside that room even, but it gave me some comfort to know that other people were indeed carrying on as normal. *Maybe there would be hope for me too one day in the future?*

Despite all the healthcare assistant's efforts over a number of hours, we had still had no joy with the feeding and we made the decision to switch to formula-feeding, hopefully as a temporary measure while I learnt to breastfeed him properly. I was heartbroken. I felt I was depriving Jacob of his basic care. Hardly anyone I knew had formula-fed and I had so badly wanted to feed the natural way. Some areas of society would have us believe that formula milk is the equivalent of pumping poison into our babies!

'Breast is best.'

'Babies should be exclusively breastfed for their first six months.'

'Breastfeeding helps achieve optimum health and development in infants.'

'Exclusive breastfeeding reduces infant mortality.'

These are just some of the messages that expectant and new mums are flooded with in those early days. While I'm sure nobody would dispute their truth, there also needs to be a balance between the promotion of breastfeeding and not making already vulnerable, exhausted mums feel demonised if they are unable to. It seems like we can't catch a break at any turn.

I was shown how to express some colostrum that was then syringed into Jacob's mouth, so at least that was some comfort. A line from the breastfeeding booklet played over and over again in my head: "Babies already know how to breastfeed. It's mothers who need to learn how to do it." I felt ashamed as I put the bottle to Jacob's lips; I had failed him at the first hurdle and was possibly putting his health and his future development in jeopardy. I was still determined that I would breastfeed in the longer term; formula-feeding had never even been on my radar throughout the pregnancy. It just wasn't the "done thing" amongst my friends. I didn't want anyone to know I wasn't breastfeeding yet, so I would try to hide the bottle whenever somebody came into the room.

All the while, visitors came and went – my parents, my sister, my auntie and uncle. I knew I had to pretend that everything was okay with me, so I went through the motions, talking about the birth and our plans for the next few days. By the time my auntie and uncle visited, I was mortified to realise that the sheets I was lying on had not yet been changed in the time I had been there. I had been told to keep clean and dry to avoid infection, yet I was sitting in heavily soiled sheets that were covered in blood and various other postpartum bodily fluids that tend to appear.

Michael and I asked for the sheets to be changed several times, but to no avail. In the end, after my auntie and uncle had left, I ended up stripping the bed myself and taking the sheets out into the corridor.

'Please,' I almost begged one of the nurses. 'Can I have clean sheets?'

Having the dirty sheets thrown at their feet meant that the staff couldn't ignore me anymore, and they went off to fetch me some clean ones. Michael and I had to put the new bedding on ourselves (despite me really being in no fit state physically to do this, having just *given birth*), but I was beyond caring by that point.

It felt wonderful to have a clean bed to lie on once again. The small things make such a big difference when feeling so vulnerable post-birth!

Although we had switched to formula-feeding, it became apparent that Jacob wasn't latching onto the bottle either. Hours went by and the lovely, patient healthcare assistant called for more help as Jacob became hungrier and hungrier. Eventually, he was examined by a doctor who said that he had such a build-up of rubbish on his chest that he wasn't able to feed properly. From then onwards, Jacob was propped up in his crib so that he could breathe more easily and hopefully start to clear the rubbish away. When Jacob took his first full feed from a bottle late in the evening, the relief was instant and immense.

By this time, we had been told that Michael was welcome to stay overnight with me, so he suggested I get some sleep while he looked after Jacob, now that he was able to be fed from a bottle. I was so relieved that Michael was going to be with me. If nothing else, at least he would be able to see the struggles I'd been having with his own eyes.

As I lay down to sleep, I heard a commotion out in the corridor. The sad and desperate voice of a young lady was screaming, 'I'm going to kill my baby!'

Michael poked his head out into the corridor and saw two doctors running towards the woman. One of the doctors injected her with something (most likely a sedative), and things quietened down immediately.

Her voice still haunts my dreams from time to time. The most frightening thing is, at that moment in time, I didn't blame her for having such an abhorrent urge. The last thing I wanted to do was hurt Jacob, but the way I was feeling, I could almost see how someone could feel that way. Once you reach that level of exhaustion, your thoughts stop being rational and any sense of reality is gone. Nothing seems real anymore, so you think it probably wouldn't matter if something awful happens. Nothing can affect someone who is numb to normal emotional responses.

*

At this point, I had gone almost 72 hours without sleep and was hallucinating badly. I was having conversations with people who weren't there.

'Your baby's lovely,' they kept saying.

'Thanks,' I would reply. 'It's a little girl, called Jacob.'

I was repeatedly referring to Jacob as "she", and genuinely believed he was a girl. I had no idea what day of the week it was, what time it was, or how long I'd been in hospital. It could have been days, it could have been months.

Michael and I both tried to tell the staff, but we were brushed off to begin with.

'Well, you won't get much sleep with a newborn,' we were told, time and time again.

'No,' I tried to tell them, 'I don't mean I'm not getting much sleep. I mean I haven't had even a minute's sleep in three days now.'

But it was to no avail. I felt desperate – here we were asking for help, only to be told there was none. I honestly couldn't see how I would ever sleep again.

Eventually, at about two o'clock in the morning, Michael insisted I see a doctor. When the doctor came, he reluctantly agreed to give me something to help me sleep, and made us promise that Michael would be in sole care of Jacob while I was under the effects of the medication.

'We have another lady on the main maternity ward,' he said. 'I gave her sleeping medication earlier on, then she tried to pick up her baby and dropped him onto the floor.'

I wondered why he was telling me this. Was he wanting me to change my mind and say I wouldn't take the pills after all? Is it really fair to expect that of someone who is suffering so acutely? While it was an awful thing to have happened, I didn't know this lady or her baby, so it was nothing to me. I wasn't capable of empathy in that moment.

I swallowed the pills gratefully, not stopping to ask any questions about what they were or any side effects. As long as they made me sleep, I didn't care.

I lay in bed, willing myself to drop off, but the pills wouldn't work. I was completely wired and hallucinating – everywhere I looked, I could see terrible, frightening faces of people who, while not there physically, absolutely were there in my head. These were the people from the horror movies, the worst of the worst nightmares. They were coming to harm me and there was nothing I could do about it. I was on constant high alert, waiting for the people in the room to either come and kill me or leave me be.

'Where is she?' I kept asking Michael.

'Who?'

'The baby.'

In my mind, Jacob was a girl, but she wasn't mine. I was supposed to be looking after her for somebody else, but why weren't they coming back for her? *Don't they know I need to sleep? I shouldn't have to be watching someone else's baby like this; they should be doing it themselves. I don't even know this baby's name, for goodness' sake!*

These hallucinations were exhausting and would not let me rest. Eventually, I did manage about three hours' sleep. I tried to see this as a positive – and, for now at least, some of the hallucinations had been staved off.

When the morning broke, Michael went home to get a few hours' rest. The nurses told me that I would be able to go home that day, so I spent some time getting my things together in anticipation. I wandered down the corridor to get some breakfast and was once again told off for leaving Jacob in the room on his own. I just couldn't see any problem with it – okay, so he might get stolen, but then at least I might be able to get some uninterrupted rest. That was how muddled my thoughts and feelings were at that time. The nurses either didn't seem to notice I was acting strangely, didn't have the time to deal with it, or just didn't care and wanted me gone so they could have my room back. I hope it was the first one.

Michael returned after lunch and we were shown how to bathe Jacob. He also had his newborn checks on his eyes, heart, hips, and testicles, which were thankfully all normal. After my three hours of sleep, I felt just about strong enough to give breastfeeding another try, and this time there was a nurse available to sit with me and show me how to do it properly. I could tell straightaway that the latch was perfect this time – it was such a unique, wonderful feeling, like nothing I have experienced before or since. It was something very primal, something instinctive. My baby and I just fitted together in that moment and for the first time since Jacob's birth, I felt some kind of a connection to him. I fed him for 45 minutes straight that afternoon. I only wish I'd known then that it would be our first and last proper feed. If I had, I would have tried to remember every small detail, every suckle, every stroke of his cheek. Most of all, I would have got Michael to take a photograph.

A lady from the local community breastfeeding team came to my room just after we had finished feeding.

'Are you breastfeeding or formula-feeding?'

I felt proud as I told her I would be breastfeeding. I was no longer one of the formula-feeders; I was now part of a more elite group: the middle-class yummy mummies with their Bugaboos and designer changing-bags. (And yes, I realise how ridiculous that is.) She arranged to give me a call the following day to see how I was getting on and to arrange to come and visit us at home to offer any guidance or support I needed.

After waiting for the whole day, we were finally discharged at a quarter past ten that night. In hindsight, I wish we had pushed to stay overnight, as walking out into a cold October darkness was a huge shock to the system after pretty much being cooped up in one dark room for days. What's more, it was a shock that I didn't need.

I stared up at the rain-sodden sky as we walked back to the car and was suddenly terrified.

What the hell have we done?

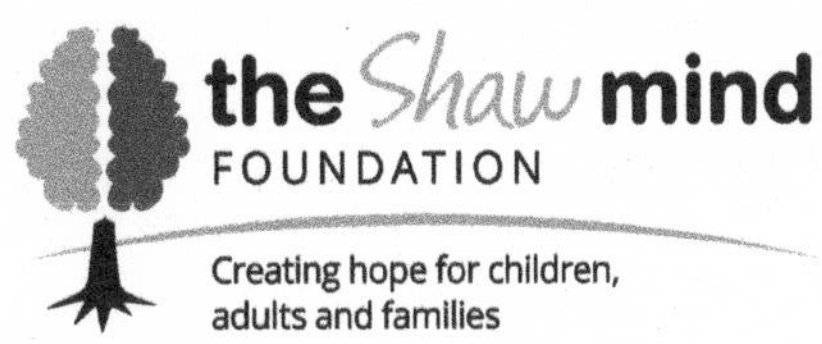

Additional copies of the tables from this book can be downloaded from the Trigger Press website.
Please visit the link below:

www.triggerpublishing.com

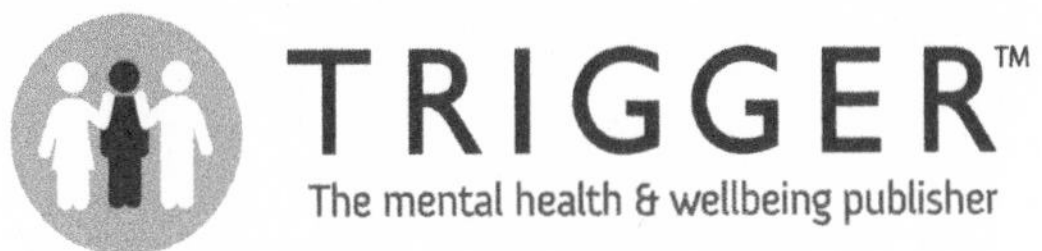

www.triggerpublishing.com

Trigger Press is a publishing house devoted to opening conversations about mental health. We tell the stories of people who have suffered from mental illnesses and recovered, so that others may learn from them.

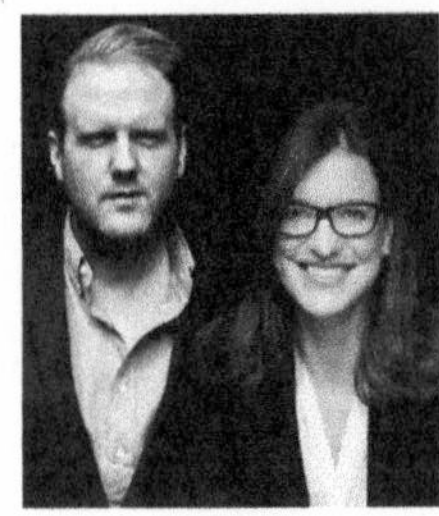

Adam Shaw is a worldwide mental health advocate and philanthropist. Now in recovery from mental health issues, he is committed to helping others suffering from debilitating mental health issues through the global charity he co-founded, The Shaw Mind Foundation. www.shawmindfoundation.org

Lauren Callaghan (CPsychol, PGDipClinPsych, PgCert, MA (hons), LLB (hons), BA), born and educated in New Zealand, is an innovative industry-leading psychologist based in London, United Kingdom. Lauren has worked with children and young people, and their families, in a number of clinical settings providing evidence based treatments for a range of illnesses, including anxiety and obsessional problems. She was a psychologist at the specialist national treatment centres for severe obsessional problems in the UK and is renowned as an expert in the field of mental health, recognised for diagnosing and successfully treating OCD and anxiety related illnesses in particular. In addition to appearing as a treating clinician in the critically acclaimed and BAFTA award-winning documentary *Bedlam*, Lauren is a frequent guest speaker on mental health conditions in the media and at academic conferences. Lauren also acts as a guest lecturer and honorary researcher at the Institute of Psychiatry Kings College, UCL.

Please visit the link below:

www.triggerpublishing.com

Join us and follow us ...

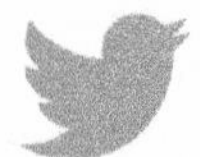

@triggerpub

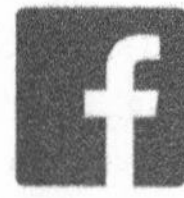

Search for us on Facebook